WHAT COLOR IS YOUR DIET?

David Heber, M.D., Ph.D.

WHAT COLOR IS YOUR DIET?

THE 7 COLORS OF HEALTH

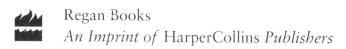

Regan Books
An Imprint of HarperCollins *Publishers*

WHAT COLOR IS YOUR DIET? Copyright © 2001 by David Heber, M.D., Ph.D.
All rights reserved. Printed in the United States of America. No part of this book may be
used or reproduced in any manner whatsoever without written permission except in the
case of brief quotations embodied in critical articles and reviews. For information
address HarperCollins Publishers Inc., 10 East 53rd Street, New York, NY 10022.

HarperCollins books may be purchased for educational, business, or sales promotional
use. For information please write: Special Markets Department, HarperCollins
Publishers Inc., 10 East 53rd Street, New York, NY 10022.

FIRST EDITION

Printed on acid-free paper

Library of Congress Cataloging-in-Publication Data has been applied for.

ISBN 0-06-039379-3

01 02 03 04 05   RRD   10 9 8 7 6 5 4 3 2 1

To my family, my patients,

my friends, my steadfast supporters,

and anyone faced with eating what is put in front of them

and wondering what they can do about it

to improve their health

This book is not intended to replace medical advice or be a substitute for a physician. If you are sick or suspect you are sick, you should see a physician. If you are taking a prescription medication, you should never change your diet or the amount that you exercise (for better or worse) without consulting your physician, because such changes will affect the metabolism of that prescription drug.

Prevention will always be the best medicine. However, prevention can only be undertaken by the individual, and that includes eating correctly and exercising routinely. This is the foundation of a healthy lifestyle.

Although this book is about diet and exercise, the author and publisher expressly disclaim responsibility for any adverse effects arising from following the advice in this book without appropriate medical supervision.

Contents

Introduction   **xiii**

Colors Protect Your Body from Oxygen Damage · Junk Foods and Junk Diets · Take Charge of Your Diet Again · Fruits and Vegetables Add Nutrition and Subtract Calories · What's New About Fruits and Vegetables · Why This Book? · Learn Why You Are Doing This · My Personal Reasons for Wanting to Help You

I Colorize Your Diet

1 What Color Is Your Diet?   **3**

From Beige to Rainbows of Color · DNA and the Language of Four Bases · DNA and Genes · DNA Damage and What You Can Do About It · DNA Protection from the Diet · DNA Damage and Common Diseases · Lessons from Around the World · The DNA Code and the Color Code for Fruits and Vegetables · Controlling Overeating by Redesigning Your Diet · Coloring Your Diet with the Color Code · Genes and Diets: Why Are You at Risk? · Putting It All Together to Colorize Your Diet

2 Colorizing Your Diet   13

Matching Your Calories to Your Body · Matching Your Protein Intake to Your Body · Controlling Your Fat Intake · Fruits and Vegetables and Spices: Your Garden Pharmacy · The Color Code System for Fruits and Vegetables · Why This Is Not a "One Sentence" Diet Plan · The Foods You Pick Are the Foods You Eat · Color Code Diet Plans

3 Using the Color Code   39

If You Don't Buy It, You Can't Eat It · The Clean Sweep · Trimming Away Excess Fat · Redesigning Your Dinner Plate · The Heart of the Colorful Kitchen: Fruits and Vegetables · Color Code Foods Made Easy · Spices and Other Staples · Super Soy Protein Solutions · Sometimes You Feel Like a Nut · Filling Up with Air-Popped Popcorn · Color Code Recipes · Shopping List for a Week of Color

4 Traveling and Dining with Your Color Code   75

Avoiding the Big-Plate Special · Focus on Fat: Restaurant Style · The International Color Code · Order What You Want · Traveling with Your Color Code · Eating at Family Gatherings and on Holidays

5 Getting Off the Couch   86

Building Muscle · Fitting in Fitness · Get Hooked on a Healthy Addiction · Circuit Training for Building and Maintaining Muscle · Planning Your Foods Before and After Exercise

6 Supplements: Pills and Foods for Health   93

The Core Group of Vitamins and Minerals · Echinacea · Chinese Red Yeast Rice · Feverfew · Saw Palmetto · Ginseng · Garlic · Ginkgo Bilob · Kava Kava · Valerian · St. John's Wort

7 Discovering the World of Plant Foods   106

Broadening a Boring Diet · Try Some New Fruits and Vegetables · You Ain't Seen Nothin' Yet · Herbs and Spices You Can Grow or Collect · Growing Your Own Herbs · Pepper, Chili Peppers, and Chili Oils · Be a Little Bit Nuts · Just a Beginning

**8 The Fifteen Most Common Myths
    About Nutrition   123**

Why Is There So Much Confusion About Food? · All You Need to Do to
Lose Weight Is to Eat Less of Your Favorite Foods · Cutting Out All the
Fat in Your Diet Is All You Need to Do · Cutting Out All the Sugar in Your
Diet Is All You Need to Do · Eating Too Few Calories Will Cause Your
Body to Go into Starvation Mode and You Will Stop Losing Weight ·
High-Protein Diets Cause Ketosis, Which Reduces Hunger · All You Need
to Do Is Exercise to Lose Weight, Since Diets Don't Work · You Get All the
Vitamins and Minerals You Need by Eating the Basic Four Food Groups ·
Carrots and Bananas Are Fattening · Peanut Butter Is a Good Source of
Protein · Pork Is the Other White Meat · Eating More Margarine and
Vegetable Oils Lowers Cholesterol · Eating Salmon Will Lower Cholesterol
Levels · Shrimp Will Raise Cholesterol Levels · Cheese Crackers Are a
Good Source of Calcium · Frozen Vegetables Aren't as Good as Fresh

II Colorize for Optimum Wellness

9 How DNA Damage Leads to Disease   137

Common Diseases Have Common Causes · Oxygen Radicals Lead to
Damaged Cells, Dead Cells, and Cancer · Smoking Produces Oxygen
Radicals and Eats Up Antioxidants · Pollution and Oxygen Damage to
DNA · Why Is DNA Damage So Deadly? · The Antioxidant Defense
System · The Common Thread of Inflammation · Diet and Inflammation:
Hints from Aspirin · How Fruits and Vegetables Protect Your DNA

**10 The Surprising Fat Cell: Much More
     Than a Bag of Fat   148**

Fat Cells Act Like White Blood Cells · The Best-Laid Plans of Mice and
Men · Is Leptin the Cure for Fat? · Leptin Is Part of the Immune System ·
Fat Cells Store Colorful Chemical Protectors · Fat Cells, Fat Cells—
Everywhere · How Many Fat Cells Do You Need? · Fat Cells That Won't
Go Away · Fat Cells Are Serious Business · Small Babies Sometimes
Make Fat Grown-ups · Humans Are Well-Adapted to Starvation, Not

Overnutrition · Fat Can Make You Sexy · Fat Can Keep You Fertile · Ancient Advantage Becomes Modern Disease · How Much Body Fat Is the Right Amount? · How the Color Code Helps

11   Heart Disease, Cholesterol, and Your DNA   157

What Is Cholesterol? · The Making of a Heart Attack · Genes for High Cholesterol? · Statin Drugs and Red Yeast Rice · Apolipoprotein B · Homocysteine · Fibrinogen, Inflammation, and Infection · The Benefits of Plant Foods · Heart Disease Can Be Prevented

12   Cancer Is a DNA Disease   171

Cancer Is a Disease of Civilization · How Cancer Grows and Spreads · High Risk, Low Risk: The Roles of Diet and Environment · The Transformation of a Pre-Carcinogen into a Carcinogen · Slowing Cancer Growth with Calorie Restriction · Oxidation, Antioxidants, and Cancer · Why Tobacco Doesn't Always Cause Cancer · Dietary Patterns That Increase Cancer Risk · Modulating Immune Function with Pro-Biotic Bacteria · The Importance of Early Detection

**13   Aging, Sex Drive, Mental Function,
        and Your DNA   186**

Why Do We Age? · We Are Living Longer Than Ever · Theories of Aging · Telomere Shortening · Cellular Checkpoints and DNA Mutations · Calorie Restriction Retards Aging · Antioxidants Slow Aging · Extra Muscle, Not Fat, May Be an Advantage · Calcium, Vitamin D, and Vitamin B_{12} Supplements · Living Longer and Feeling Better · Maintaining Your Vision · Prevent Thinning Bones and Fractures · Some Plant Estrogens May Help · You Have to Fall Over to Break Your Hip · Keep Your Sex Drive · Maintain Your Memory · Alzheimer's Disease and Antioxidants · Common Denominators

**III   Your Genes and Foods: Yesterday,
        Today, and Tomorrow**

14   Gene-Diet Imbalance and Damage to DNA   201

Balanced Nutrition in Early Life · After the Breast · Eating When You're Not Hungry · Eating Is Not Dining Anymore · Tastes Great, Less Filling

• The Battle for Your Taste Buds • The Science of Taste Modification • The Enlarging American Plate • Dopamine and Food "Addictions" • Serotonin, the Pleasure Hormone • Trigger Foods and Stress • Binge-Eating Disorder • Overeating and the Risk of Diabetes, Heart Disease, and Cancer • What You Can Learn from a Rat • Fat Cells and Your Set-Point • Why Women Are Fatter Than Men • The Big Picture

15 Cultural Evolution and the Loss of Eden   213

A Brief Early History of Humans on Earth • Mankind Explores Earth • One Big, Happy Family? • Pop's Y Chromosomes and Mom's Mitochondria • High Priests and Invading Armies • Genetic Evidence of a Lost Tribe in Africa • Moving Up the Nile River • Prescription Drugs, Plant Foods, and Genes • The Coevolution of Animal and Plant Life • The Modern Jungle Is a TV commercial • Man Disrupts the Gardens of Eden • The Emergence of Agriculture • The Ice Age and Mutated Plant Foods • Plant and Crop Domestication • From Discovery of a New World to Fusion Cuisine • Early American Foods • The Midwest Takes Over • The USDA Pyramid: Horse, Camel, or Prescription for Obesity?

16 Food Evolution and Agricultural Economics   228

The History of the Potato Chip • Don't Take Away My Doughnuts! • Red-Hot Dachshunds and Salisbury Steaks • Ketchup or Catsup? • The Invention of Peanut Butter • Never on Sundae • What's the Point? • The Hunter-Gatherer Dietary Guidelines Committee • Ancient Agriculture versus Modern Food Production and Marketing • The Culinary Melting Pot • Restoring Variety to Our Diets • The 1950s Pleasantville Diet Creates Diet-Book Best-Sellers • Vitamin Supplements and Weight-Loss Industries Thrive • Academia and the Food Industry versus Government • The Trouble with the RDA • The Politics of Nutrition • Choosing New Foods Is Still Possible • The Story of Olestra, the Fat-Free Fat • Agriculture Responds to Consumers • The Consumer Is King • The Prevention Prescription Is Optimizing Our Diets

**Appendix 1: Determining Your Calorie and Protein
                Requirements   247**

Appendix 2: Tools   **251**

Recommended Reading and References   **253**

Acknowledgments   **259**

Index   **261**

Introduction

What color is your diet? Is it beige or white? Most Americans eat far too few foods with any color in them. Studies show that the average total intake of fruits and vegetables is about three servings a day, with a serving being a half cup of cooked vegetables or a cup of raw vegetables or a piece of fruit. That boils down to two vegetables and a fruit. If those three servings consist of iceberg lettuce, French fries, and a little ketchup for color, you are in big trouble!

For most Americans the centerpiece of their diet is grains (including bread) and meat. A big hunk of steak or chicken is the main focus of the meal, and about 10 percent of Americans eat no fruits and vegetables at all.

While almost every food has something to recommend it, many are virtually devoid of the powerful colorful chemicals that can protect your genes, your vision, and your heart and can reduce inflammation in your body to help prevent common forms of cancer and other diseases that go with aging.

Colors Protect Your Body
from Oxygen Damage

Foods have colors because they contain chemicals called "phytonutrients" ("phyto" means plant) that can absorb light in the visible spectrum. They do this because they contain a certain type of chemical bond,
called a "double bond," between carbon atoms, a bond that is actually a
cloud of electrons capable of absorbing potentially damaging, renegade
electrons circling activated oxygen atoms called "oxygen radicals."
These radicals aren't threatening to burn down the administration building at the local college, but they do burnlike damage to many parts of the
living cells in your body, including damaging DNA, the key chemicals
in your genes. While not all the health-promoting chemicals in plants
absorb color, enough of them do so that it makes sense to get as much
color and as much in the way of different colors into your diet.

Junk Foods and Junk Diets

I don't mean to pick on any single food. There are no pure junk foods,
but when you put enough weak foods together, you have a junk diet. It's
not only what we are eating too much of—calories in the form of added
sugar and fat in high-fat, high-sweet treats—but also what we are not
eating enough of—colorful fruits and vegetables. One inescapable property of your diet is that there is only a limited volume of foods that you
can reasonably eat each day. Therefore, when you add something that
has less calories per bite, you push out something else with more calories
per bite. Fruits and vegetables not only have fewer calories per bite, but
more nutrition per bite than the high-fat foods they replace.

Take Charge of Your Diet Again

If you feel your diet is out of control, this book is for you. High-fat, high-
sweet foods sneak into your diet calories that you never intended to consume. I am not against sugar and fat—they are everywhere. Even fruits
and vegetables have some sugar and fat, but it is not nearly at the level of
the extra sugar, oil, and salt used to jack up the taste of snack foods so

that you will buy more and more. As you add fruits and vegetables to your diet, replacing other snack foods, you will reeducate your palate to enjoy the freshness of real foods again.

Fruits and Vegetables Add Nutrition and Subtract Calories

Adding fruits and vegetables to your diet can replace refined grains such as breads, pastas, cakes, and pastries as well as high-fat meats that bring with them extra calories you simply can't burn off. If you have been struggling with your weight, you are not alone. In fact, one of every two Americans is overweight or obese. It is time for you to do something about your diet—but what?

What's New About Fruits and Vegetables

Everyone knows, or should know, that fruits and vegetables are healthy. So what is new and different about this book? A piece of iceberg lettuce or a white potato is not the same as a red tomato, an orange carrot, or a blue blueberry.

Each colored fruit or vegetable provides a unique benefit to the diet, so you don't want to eat only fruits and vegetables of a single color. Each fruit or vegetable—whether red, yellow, green, or purple—provides a benefit that is sometimes concentrated in a particular part of the body or uses a specific pathway within your body to provide its healthful effects. You will learn how to add different fruits and vegetables to your diet by using my Color Code, which is based on the specific beneficial substances that help to prevent the common diseases that affect many of us as we get older.

- ❖ You will learn how adding fruits and vegetables to your diet can reduce calorie intake while increasing nutritional value so that you lose weight and keep it off in a healthy way.
- ❖ You will learn which fruits and vegetables can help prevent the commonest cause of preventable blindness (macular degeneration) in the United States

- ❖ You will learn which fruits and vegetables can help prevent strokes.
- ❖ You will learn which fruits and vegetables may help prevent the commonest forms of cancer, including breast, prostate, and colon cancer.
- ❖ You will learn how fruits and vegetables can protect, in four different ways, your DNA, the critical material in your genes, from damage.
- ❖ You will learn how fruits and vegetables can protect your body from inflammation—one root cause of heart disease and common forms of cancer.
- ❖ You will learn how to combine the fruits and vegetables with fiber, protein, and certain key vitamins and minerals for optimum health, based on your body using personalized formulas for protein, calories, and fat.

Why This Book?

Most diet books start with a gimmick such as reducing or eliminating fat from the diet. This can result in too little protein and a loss of muscle. Other books encourage diets that are high-protein and high-fat and have little or no sugar or refined carbohydrates. This can eliminate the good carbohydrates such as fruits and vegetables.

This book is different in organizing your whole diet, starting with fruits and vegetables as the base and then customizing your calorie and protein needs to your body. The amount of lean versus fat tissue in your body, not your height or weight, determines your calorie needs.

The amount of lean tissue in your body also determines how much protein you will need. You will be given personalized prescriptions for your daily protein and calorie needs. Then, using this framework, you will learn about the benefits of spices and herbs, vitamins and minerals. By tailoring the diet to your personal needs, this book will provide you with the healthiest possible diet, and one that will help you lose weight and keep it off.

Learn Why You Are Doing This

Unlike many diet books, once you learn what to do you will also learn why you are doing it. Some people just want to know what to do, and trust that it will work. However, if you also want to know why, then this book is for you. In this book you will learn about human genetics and how diet interacts with your DNA. DNA is short for a chemical called "deoxyribonucleic acid," which makes up the human genome—the personal code that defines who you are in every cell of your body. It is damage to the DNA that is the root cause of cancer and many other common diseases. In this book you will learn how this happens and how the chemicals found in fruits and vegetables can protect your DNA from damage.

You will also learn why this diet makes sense. Man evolved on a plant-based diet fifty thousand years ago, and our modern diet developed only over the last fifty to a hundred years. Our modern diet is out of balance with our genes, and in this book you will learn how to restore the balance that nature intended.

My Personal Reasons for Wanting to Help You

My purpose in writing this book was to translate my knowledge of the role your diet can play in providing you with optimum health. I have been a practicing medical doctor and a physician-scientist specializing in nutrition for the past twenty years. I established the Division of Clinical Nutrition at UCLA in 1983 and the UCLA Center for Human Nutrition in 1996. I am also a professor of medicine and public health at UCLA, where I teach both in the medical school and the college. My preparation for an exciting career in nutrition included an undergraduate degree in chemistry from UCLA, where I spent three summers in the laboratory of a Nobel Prize winner. I received my medical degree from Harvard Medical School, where I spent two years working in the endocrine laboratory of a renowned scientist who was studying hormone secretion. I completed my internship at Beth Israel Hospital in Boston, and completed an internal medicine residency at Harbor General Hospital in Torrance, California, where I also worked for three years as a research fellow in endocrinology. I received a Ph.D. in physiology from UCLA for research on a tiny protein that controls reproduction in men and women by acting on a specialized area of the brain. At the end of my fellowship at Harbor General Hospital, I began a career in nutrition research, teaching, and patient care, and I joined the UCLA faculty. I still see patients, teach, and conduct research in nutrition in three fields—obesity, cancer prevention and treatment, and herbal supplements.

I have also written this book because I believe we are at a critical juncture in American medicine, where something will have to change. In the next century I believe medicine must emphasize prevention through health education and changes in the food supply, rather than by simply treating diseases after the damage has been done. Many medical authorities speak about disease as if nutrition was completely irrelevant. Eat whatever you want and high-tech medicine will cure your diseases after the damage has occurred. I take a different approach. With the simple changes in diet described in this book, you will be able to influence your health. Every revolution starts with individuals—in this case, it is you! Join me on a fascinating journey as you learn how to add to your diet a family of colors that will help protect your DNA and prevent the most common diseases from threatening your health and longevity.

COLORIZE
YOUR DIET

What Color Is Your Diet?

There is a tradition that colors our diets beige. Discovered in the Fertile Crescent, beige grains such as wheat provided a reliable source of calories—but at a price. Egyptians ate a beige, grain-based diet in ancient times, and when Egyptian mummies were unearthed they demonstrated remarkable evidence of arthritis, diabetes, and cancer. Early farmers were also shorter than hunter-gatherers, due to the nutritional deficiencies of their grain-based diet compared to the colorful diversity of the hunter-gatherer's diet. During the Roman Empire grains were exported from Egypt to Rome to be fed to the lower classes to keep them from rioting. Are fast foods playing a similar role in our modern society? We have a grain-based diet that includes corn oil, corn sugar, and corn-fed beef, all of which are inexpensive and available twenty-four hours a day. Our pets eat a grain-based diet and suffer from cancer, diabetes, and other diseases of man. Even our laboratory rats get a beige-pelleted chow diet and suffer from a high rate of obesity and spontaneous tumors as they age.

Eating is a pleasure, and we have voted with our dollars for a beige diet of French fries, burgers, and cheese. The only problem with the diet we love is that it doesn't fit our genes, which evolved over eons in a plant-based, hunter-gatherer diet with half the fat, no dairy products, no processed foods, no refined sugars, no alcohol, and no tobacco. Our closest animal relatives, gorillas and chimpanzees, choose a richly diverse selection of plant foods based on color, size, texture, and taste. Today, in places such as New Guinea, we can still find hunter-gatherer populations who eat more than eight hundred varieties of plant foods. Americans eat fewer than twenty different fruits and vegetables, and most Americans eat only three servings of these a day. Adding foods is easier than taking them away, so we will start with a simple addition of fruits and vegetables to help protect your genes from being damaged.

From Beige to Rainbows of Color

Habits, whether good or bad, are familiar and pleasant and shield us from the storm of everyday stress. As stress has increased in our lives, so has stress eating. The rise of steak houses, take-out restaurants, and the continuing popularity of familiar burger-and-fries fast-food restaurants attest to the staying power of stress-release eating. You may know deep down that eating the way you are is not good, but you don't know how to change. If you are ready to change the way you are eating to improve your health, for whatever reason, this book is for you. I wrote this book to simplify much of the confusing information out there about diet so that you can change now. It's no good continuing to eat unhealthy food until the last juror comes back on every scientific study. You can't wait until every naysayer agrees. By then we'll all be dead. Now is the time to change your eating habits or get them tuned up to maximize your health and longevity.

The fact of the matter is that there is a solid foundation of knowledge in nutrition and exciting new breakthroughs in human genetics and disease that tell us loud and clear: Eat a colorful diet. My job is to translate information from scientific jargon into understandable, everyday English while maintaining its essential truth.

DNA and the Language of Four Bases

DNA is found in every cell of your body as part of a long chain of four different but closely related units called "DNA bases." There are four different bases, A, T, G, and C, which form a biological alphabet that the body can read to program the production of specific proteins.

The program for each protein is called a "gene." Imagine the bases making up each gene as links between two mirror-image strands of a double helix that can be unzipped and can dictate the exact sequence of these bases on another strand of DNA. Certain bases pair up with other bases, so A always goes with T and G always goes with C. It is this language and the integrity of the DNA zipper that makes the miracle of cell reproduction possible. Cells involved in producing a new human being consist of single strands from two different individuals, so you inherit traits from both your mother and your father. The simple DNA code of four bases continuing through twenty-three different pairs of bodies called "chromosomes" makes up a total of 4 billion such letters to form your personal genetic code. Every time a cell divides, which happens every few hours for cells on the tongue and in the intestine, the DNA must unzip and rezip perfectly. Errors are sometimes made, and these are then repaired. However, as we age there is an accumulation of damage to DNA, much of it harmless. But on occasion, the damage programs the development of cancer, heart disease, or diabetes.

The Color Code is designed to minimize this damage by teaching you to eat protective foods and dietary supplements within a healthy diet.

DNA and Genes

When translated, the information found in DNA provides the text that sets the stage for the development of all your physical and behavioral attributes, including hair, nails, internal organs, bones, brain, personality, and the sperm or egg cells necessary for passing your genes on to the next generation. We know that over 90 percent of our DNA is not actually coding for the production of proteins but is thought to be concerned with regulating how our DNA is used. So damage to DNA can affect how genes are turned on and off, and this process can influence the development of a number of diseases, including common forms of cancer.

DNA Damage and What You Can Do About It

How is DNA damaged in our bodies? The answer is oxygen. Oxygen first formed in our atmosphere hundreds of millions of years ago as bacteria harnessed the energy in sunlight to make energy. This oxygen, which makes up 20 percent of the volume of the air we breathe, when exposed to heat and light becomes an oxygen radical. An oxygen radical is much like bleach, due to the presence of an unpaired subatomic particle called an "electron." This electron roves around looking for targets to react with, and it can alter proteins, fats, sugars, and the DNA in your cells. In response to the hazards of oxygen, plants developed the wonderful rainbow of colors we associate with red strawberries, deep green broccoli, and orange carrots.

All of these colored substances are in the plants to protect them from oxygen in the atmosphere. They appear colored to our eyes because their chemical structure absorbs visible light. The chemical property that enables them to absorb light also makes it possible for them to neutralize the electrons that can harm your DNA. If you grow fruit-bearing plants in poor soil that causes them to be pale, you will notice black spots on the fruit and leaves where the plants have been burned by the oxygen in the air. If you cut open an apple, it turns brown within a minute or two of exposure to the air. The red skin of the apple protects it from the damaging effects of oxygen. When we eat the red skin of an apple, we take in those same colored substances, and they help us internally protect our DNA.

DNA Protection from the Diet

By the time modern man evolved, some fifty to a hundred thousand years ago, we had come to depend on the colored substances in fruits and vegetables to protect our cells from damage. While we have systems in our bodies that make substances that protect our DNA, many, such as the gene to make vitamin C, were lost during evolution simply because they were no longer necessary given the abundance of vitamin C in our ancient diets. Some of the colored substances, such as the orange color in carrots, are stored in our fat, while other chemicals, such as those in broccoli, stimulate our cells to produce proteins that protect our DNA. Many of the protective substances found in plant foods are broken down, and we can find only about 20 percent of the amount eaten excreted in our urine. However, in the process of being broken down, these phytonutrients send a signal to our DNA to produce specific proteins, called "enzymes," that can break down both these phytonutrients and some

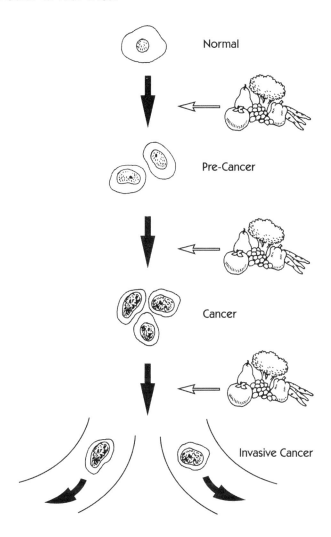

Phytochemicals Block the Cancer Process

toxins produced in our cells or taken in from our diet. As you can imagine, only those toxins that have chemical structures in common with the phytonutrient in a particular fruit or vegetable are detoxified.

So it makes sense to take in as diverse a group of plant foods as possible. These enzymes, which evolved to break down phytonutrients, also protect our bodies from the chemicals found in drugs, from aspirin to the most potent antibiotic. The fact that drinking grapefruit juice can affect how your body breaks down the most widely prescribed cholesterol-lowering drugs proves this point. When taken at usual doses, the blood levels of the drug are found to be twice as high after drinking double-strength grapefruit juice for three days. There is an enzyme on the surface of the small intestine whose production is inhibited by chemicals in the grapefruit juice. This type of interaction of chemicals in grapefruit juice with your genes is an example of how diet can powerfully affect the body's enzyme systems. There are many other examples mentioned later, but the point is that these enzyme changes also can protect your body from chemicals in the diet or the environment.

DNA Damage and Common Diseases

As we age, our DNA protection systems become less effective and we generate more oxygen in our cells. Damage to our DNA piles up, and some of the changes in our genes lead to heart disease, cancer, and Alzheimer's disease. Obesity, which affects one out of every three Americans, stimulates the oxygen damage of DNA as well. The good news is that you can change your diet in ways that will protect your DNA.

Lessons from Around the World

The scientific data are there from studies done all over the world, waiting for you to change what you are eating.

Here are the facts:

- ❖ The risks of common forms of cancer are reduced by 50 percent in countries where about a pound of fruits and vegetables is eaten each day.
- ❖ Virtually every disease of aging—including heart disease, diabetes, and many common forms of cancer such as breast cancer and prostate cancer—results from damage to DNA, which can be prevented by the substances found in fruits and vegetables.
- ❖ 80 to 90 percent of all cancers are not inherited, but result from the defects in DNA occurring during your lifetime from accumulated damage that could be prevented by increasing fruit and vegetable intake.

❖ Over 90 percent of all diabetes is associated with overeating and obesity (I call it "diabesity") and will account for 70 to 80 percent of all heart disease deaths in the next ten years.

❖ Damage to DNA results from excess oxygen radicals that are produced as part of our normal cell processes, but the production of oxygen radicals increases as we get older and is probably involved in Alzheimer's disease, other brain disorders, and the process of aging itself.

❖ Our bodies attempt to protect our DNA in many ways, but these protections break down as we age.

❖ Our bodies depend on chemicals found in plant foods to back up our natural DNA defense mechanisms throughout life, but this becomes more important as we age.

❖ The good news is that there is something you can do.

The DNA Code and the Color Code for Fruits and Vegetables

Our DNA code was set down fifty thousand years ago, and so could not anticipate our diet of burgers, fries, chips, and pizza. It is the imbalance between our modern diet and the DNA laid down all those years ago that accounts for all of our major common diseases.

The beige/white diet commonly results in eating too many calories, so that half of all Americans are overweight. This is the grain of truth in the diet philosophy that maintains that carbohydrates cause obesity. By overeating we also send signals to our cells to grow more quickly, increasing the likelihood of DNA damage, especially when we eat too few fruits and vegetables to counteract the natural increases in DNA damage that go along with eating too many calories. The fat cells also release substances that encourage inflammation and are a key part of the processes promoting atherosclerosis and common forms of cancer. The substances in fruits and vegetables can counteract the inflammation caused by these fat-cell signals.

The Color Code will restore to the diet what is missing in a way that will optimize protection of your cells and the genes inside these cells.

Controlling Overeating by Redesigning Your Diet

Much of your overeating may be unintentional, as you eat foods with hidden sugar and oils put there to stimulate your taste buds. I will show you how to retain the taste but get rid of the extra fat and sugar. You cannot completely avoid sugar and fat. Both of these are present in fruits and vegetables in small amounts, but you can substitute healthy fruits and vegetables for processed snack foods that have unnecessarily large amounts of added sugar and oil.

Simply removing sugar and oil from your foods is not enough. You need to eat adequate protein of the right kinds. Soy protein should make up at least one half of your total protein intake each day—and you need to take in protein with each meal. A bagel and a cup of coffee is not a healthy breakfast. You will start your day with a healthy high-fiber soy breakfast cereal or a soy protein shake and fruit. Then you will have three to six ounces of low-fat proteins such as soy meat substitutes, the white meat of chicken, the white meat of turkey, ocean fish, or seafood such as shrimp, scallops, or lobster at lunch and dinner. At lunch and dinner you will also select specific fruits and vegetables using the Color Code. If you are a large man, you may need another soy shake in midafternoon. If you are a smaller woman, you will want to have three ounces of protein at lunch and dinner without a midafternoon shake.

Coloring Your Diet with the Color Code

Now that you have cut away fat and sugar, and added protein, you need the key ingredient in your new diet—a rainbow of colorful fruits and vegetables. We all know that fruits and vegetables are healthy. That is nothing new. What is new is that these foods can be classified according to color—red, red/purple, orange, orange/yellow, green, yellow/green, and white/green—based on the specific chemicals that absorb light in the visible spectrum and thus create the different colors. These chemicals are called "phytonutrients" or "phytochemicals," and each of these colored compounds works in different ways to protect your genes and your DNA. By making sure you eat a representative of each of these seven color-coded groups of fruits and vegetables every day, you will be meeting the recommendations of many government agencies, including the National Cancer Institute, that you eat five to nine servings of fruits and vegetables every day.

You will be going further to ensure that your body has what it needs to protect your DNA. Not all fruits and vegetables are the same. The different colors indicate how they differ, but you will also be getting a group of compounds called "flavonoids," which are found throughout the Color Code, up to one gram per day, and these are levels of protection you cannot achieve simply with vitamins. As you will see, I am not against vitamins in reasonable amounts as a supplement to the diet. However, they are not an excuse for continuing to eat an unhealthy diet.

Genes and Diets: Why Are You at Risk?

Not all of us are alike. Some can smoke, drink, and eat whatever they want with no apparent harm. In this book you will learn about human genetics and why I believe so many of us will not be quite so lucky as to emerge from the American diet unscathed. For much of man's existence on earth, food was scarce. The only way to get enough calories was to eat pounds of plant foods. In some places on earth, mankind still eats a biodiverse rainbow of colored plant foods. We evolved to have genes to conserve calories so we would not starve. We also evolved genes to be able to rid our bodies of the excess phytonutrients in our ancient diet. Those hunter-gatherers who still eat this way today don't suffer from obesity, heart disease, diabetes, cancer, high blood pressure, excess stomach acid. However, if you have the most common genes, you will be susceptible to these diseases of civilization.

Putting It All Together to Colorize Your Diet

In this book you will learn how to change your diet in simple ways that will protect your DNA from damage.

❖ You will replace bland, starchy foods with colorful fruits and vegetables by using a simple Color Code system.

❖ You will replace foods with hidden vegetable oils and added refined sugar with healthy, great-tasting foods that are high in fiber and are filling.

❖ You will get adequate protein at each meal to maintain your muscles and to ensure that you are not hungry without going on an unhealthy high-fat, high-protein diet.

❖ You will learn how soy protein and green tea can protect your DNA.

❖ You will learn which vitamins, minerals, and dietary supplements can help protect your DNA.

Putting all of this together in a healthy lifestyle that includes exercise and meditation will combine to reduce the damage to your DNA, which affects aging, Alzheimer's disease, cancer, diabetes, and heart disease.

As we spread our American lifestyle and foods around the world, we are creating an epidemic of obesity and cancer. It will be decades before we understand fully how diet and lifestyle can bring on each of these common diseases, but there is enough information now to enable you to bring your diet back into balance with the conditions that influenced the development of your genes and to protect your DNA.

In the next chapter you will design your own Color Code diet.

2

Colorizing
Your Diet

The key to designing your colorful diet is to place your varied selection of fruits and vegetables from the seven different color groups listed below within a customized diet-and-exercise program. The first step in this process is determining how many calories you need. If you eat more calories than you burn, you will gain weight and trigger the depletion of the substances that protect your DNA. This occurs as the body sends messages to cells to duplicate more quickly in the presence of excess calories. This overproduction of cells, combined with the damage that occurs to your DNA in the process, is the beginning of a long road that can ultimately lead to heart disease, common forms of cancer, Alzheimer's disease, and accelerated aging.

Matching Your Calories to Your Body

You can make sure you are not in positive calorie balance by watching the portion sizes of what you eat and exercising enough to prevent weight gain. If you are gaining weight, you are eating too many calories relative to the number you are burning each day. When you first switch from the usual American diet to the Color Code diet, you may lose a few pounds since fruits and vegetables carry fewer calories per bite than breads, cakes, and pastries made from refined flour. If you want a better estimate of how many calories you should be eating, see Appendix 1, where you will learn to measure your lean body mass and calculate your basic calorie requirement based on each pound of lean body mass burning 14 calories per day.

Matching Your Protein Intake to Your Body

Your lean body mass is what is left when you subtract the weight of your fat from your total body weight. Fat doesn't require much dietary protein, but each pound of lean body mass you have requires one gram of protein per day. In the absence of adequate protein intake, you will lose protein from your muscles. During the past decades, when very low fat eating was popular, protein was eliminated, or reduced drastically, in error, as pasta and other refined carbohydrates made up the bulk of the diet.

You would be surprised by how many women I have seen who had a bagel and coffee for breakfast, a salad with no meat at lunch, and pasta with no meat at dinner. They would look very thin, but would have very low lean body mass. Even though they looked thin, they were really fat when I measured their body fat. They were also hungry all the time. They needed so few calories that they were doomed to a life of severe calorie restriction. Protein will satisfy your appetite between meals, and you should have some protein with each meal until you reach your total for the day. You don't have to eat cheese, steaks, burgers, and prime rib to get the protein you need, as advised in some popular diet plans. You can get all the protein you need, without the fat, by eating the white meat of chicken or turkey, many types of fish and other seafood, and soy protein extracted from whole soybeans drinks or soy meat substitutes. Get protein at every meal. Make it three ounces at each meal if you are a woman and six ounces if you are a man and you can skip the exact calculations.

Controlling Your Fat Intake

It's easy to be fooled about the amount of fat you are eating. At any buffet or salad bar, it is possible to get a high-fat, high-fiber meal rich in fruits and vegetables by simply dousing your salad with a heavy Thousand Island, Italian, French, or Russian dressing. Did you know that a Chinese chicken salad provides over 1,000 calories? All these different nationalities of salad dressing have one thing in common—enough extra calories to add unwanted pounds of fat to your body. Use balsamic vinegar, wine vinegar, or lemon and have a salad made with dark green and leafy lettuce, green bell pepper, red bell pepper, mushrooms, onions, and tomatoes to carry the taste. If you can afford the 140 calories per tablespoon, you would be better off adding a dash of extra-virgin olive oil or little squares of avocado to your salad for a boost in taste. Olive oil and avocados contain beneficial monounsaturated fatty acids, not the hydrogenated and polyunsaturated vegetable oils found in most salad dressings.

Fruits and Vegetables and Spices: Your Garden Pharmacy

Ancient humans would have had to eat pounds of low-fat, high-fiber fruits and vegetables to extract the valuable calories needed for survival, while modern humans can't help but get too many. Just a handful of a compact snack such as peanuts, chips, or cookies provides more calories than two cups of many vegetables, and we don't expend much energy getting from the kitchen to the couch.

Not all members of the fruit and vegetable group are alike. They have unique properties that provide combinations of substances with unique effects on human biology. For example, lycopene, found in tomatoes and tomato-based products, is concentrated in the prostate gland in men. However, lutein and zeaxanthin, found in spinach, corn, and other yellow or green leafy vegetables, are concentrated in the retina and the lens, where they are associated with a reduced risk of cataracts and macular degeneration. Therefore, simply eating five servings a day of fruits and vegetables will not guarantee that you are eating enough of the different substances needed to stimulate the metabolic pathways of genes in the different organs where fruits and vegetables have their beneficial effects. The types of foods that make up your diet's overall nutritional analysis have a tremendous influence on the beneficial chemicals, most of which are from plant foods.

I am often asked by patients what I mean by "a serving." The rule is that half a cup of a cooked vegetable or fruit or a cup of a raw vegetable or fruit constitutes one serving. You will be eating seven servings or more a day on the Color Code diet of fruits and vegetables from different color groups.

The Color Code System
for Fruits and Vegetables

Plant-eating animals naturally use color as an identifying marker of edible plants. The changing color of ripening fruits and vegetables signifies when they are at the peak of their taste and nutritive value. Many of the phytonutrients are actually the pigment molecules that lend ripe fruits and vegetables their distinctive hues.

Carotenoids are chemical compounds that absorb visible light and so determine that carrots are orange, tomatoes are red, and marigolds are yellow. Approximately seven hundred different carotenoids have been isolated from plants and animals. About fifty to sixty of these are present in a typical diet. These carotenoids are specifically broken down by the body, often during the process of absorption into the bloodstream from the small intestine. They make their way to specific tissues and organs where they have been shown to protect against the type of oxygen damage that can harm your DNA.

Because the color of a plant food can tell us so much about how it supports health, I've developed a Color Code system to help you introduce more diversity into your diet. The different colors are important because the different plant chemicals they represent have different effects on the body.

The *red group* includes tomatoes, pink grapefruit, and watermelon, all of which contain lycopene. Lycopene is more available from cooked tomato products and juices than from whole raw tomatoes, and these products are the primary sources of lycopene in our diet. So you would add red as a pasta sauce, tomato soup, tomato juice, and ketchup. As a practical matter, over 80 percent of the lycopene in the American diet comes from these tomato products.

The *red/purple group* includes grapes, red wine, grape juice, prunes, cranberries, blueberries, blackberries, strawberries, and red apples. These foods contain anthocyanins, which are powerful antioxidants that

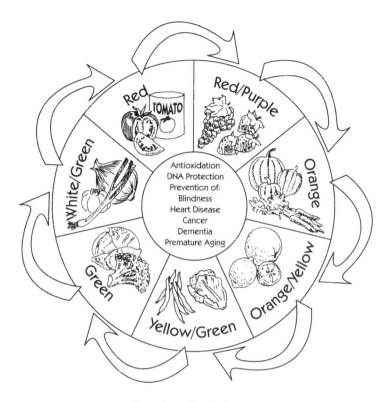

The Color Wheel of Foods

may have a beneficial effect on heart disease by inhibiting blood clot formation.

The *orange group* includes carrots, mangos, apricots, cantaloupes, pumpkin, acorn squash, winter squash, and sweet potatoes. These provide alpha- and beta-carotenes. In this group, carrots provide about half the alpha- and beta-carotene in the U.S. diet, with significant contributions from tomato products.

The *orange/yellow group* includes orange juice, oranges and tangerines, peaches, papayas, and nectarines. These provide β-cryptothanxin, a minor carotenoid that accounts for only 0.03 milligram of the 6 milligrams per day intake of all carotenoids by the average American. As a practical matter, 87 percent of β-cryptoxanthin comes from orange juice, oranges, and tangerines. Other fruits providing smaller amounts include peaches, papayas, and nectarines. These fruits obviously have other benefits and are a separate group to be used primarily to stimulate more diversity in your diet.

The *yellow/green group* includes spinach; collard, mustard, or turnip greens; yellow corn; green peas; avocado; and honeydew melon. These provide lutein and zeaxanthin as well. These carotenoids concentrate in the eye and contribute to eye health. Lower intakes have been associated with cataracts and age-related macular degeneration, the primary preventable cause of blindness in America.

The *green group* includes broccoli; Brussels sprouts; cabbage; Chinese cabbage, or bok choi; and kale. These contain sulforaphane, isothiocyanate, and indoles, which stimulate the genes in your liver to turn on the production of enzymes that break down the cancer-causing chemicals in the body.

The *white/green group* includes garlic, onions, celery, pears, white wine, endive, and chives. Plants in the onion family contain allicin, which has been shown to have antitumor effects. Foods in this group are also rich sources of flavonoids, including quercetin and kaempferol. Of all the antioxidants in fruits and vegetables, it is the flavonoids that we eat in the largest quantity, up to one gram per day. There are many flavonoid structures, and researchers in my laboratory are developing methods for measuring the evidence that flavonoids have been eaten based on their breakdown products in the urine.

Why This Is Not a
"One Sentence" Diet Plan

It is important to realize that when it comes to diets, you have to look at the whole diet rather than simply breaking it down into carbohydrates, proteins, and fats. We eat foods that contain these things. Most vegetables and protein foods contain fat, and all vegetables and fruits contain some sugar, a little protein, and a little fat. Eliminating all fats or sugars from your diet is impossible, but you can control those foods you choose. For each of the above food categories, there are desirable and undesirable foods, which are simply called proteins, carbohydrates, and fats. It is not practical to eliminate any of these from your diet, but it is a mistake to lump them all together without making any distinctions between them. You can make desirable choices that will help protect your DNA by avoiding obesity and overnutrition and taking in adequate amounts of the phytochemicals in fruits and vegetables.

Examples of Desirable and Undesirable Foods

	Undesirable	*Desirable*
Protein	Gelatin	Soy
	High-fat red meats	White poultry meat
	Whole eggs	Egg white
	Farmed salmon/trout, tuna, shrimp	
Carbohydrate	Sugar, pasta	Fruits, vegetables
	White bread	Whole grains
	Cakes, pastries	Air-popped corn
	Snack crackers	
Fat	Hydrogenated soy oil	Olive oil
	Corn oil	Avocado oil
	Cottonseed oil	
	Safflower oil	
	Margarine, mayonnaise, butter	

You won't be poisoned eating the undesirable categories above. However, I am not one of those people who believe that there are no such things as junk foods—just junk diets. There are many foods that don't promote your health, and these should not be the basis of your regular diet. If you put enough junk foods together, it becomes difficult not to have a junk diet.

The Foods You Pick Are the Foods You Eat

Our selection of foods today is determined by taste, cost, and convenience rather than by the careful selection process that humans evolved over millions of years. What was a sweet fruit hanging from a tree is now a cardboard box filled with sweetened, salted, processed, and oiled low-fiber snack foods that bear a health claim. It is now claimed that a cheese snack cracker is a good source of calcium. In ancient times there was so much calcium in the diet (about 1,600 milligrams) that we evolved to be inefficient in our absorption of it. Today, calcium supplements are necessary to be sure you are getting what you need to prevent bone loss. There are many other examples of chemicals that we once got from fruit and vegetables that we no longer get in the diet. Vitamin C is easily obtained from the diet by eating fruits and vegetables, and we lost the gene to manufacture vitamin C, unlike many other species that are not primarily fruit-eating. For other chemicals in foods, we make some in our bodies and take in some from the diet. These phytochemicals are just as important as vitamins for optimum health, but are best obtained from a wide variety of fruits and vegetables. Once you have obtained the needed fruits and vegetables and adequate protein, the remainder of your calories can come from carbohydrates and fats. Whole grain cereals and breads are preferable to refined carbohydrate foods, which are easier to eat in large quantities without feeling full. Whole grains also have other health benefits, including improving intestinal function and providing some DNA protectors in the diet.

Color Code Diet Plans

Here are some simple examples of Color Code diet plans for women and for men. If you are a small man or a tall woman, you may need to switch to the other gender's diet to get the number of calories you need to maintain your weight.

The diet plans for women contain about 1,200 to 1,400 calories per day; for men the number of calories is higher: about 1,800 to 2,000 calories per day. Most men, and some tall or large women, will want to use the higher-calorie plans. Both sample diets have the following in common:

1. They include, each day, foods from each of the seven color groups in the Color Code system.
2. They include protein at each meal, and aim for some soy protein in the diet every day.
3. They include whole grains for fiber and taste enhancers as needed within the total calories in the meal plan.

Here is one week on the Color Code diet, with the color groups noted so that you can see how easy it is to make your seven servings each day. Recipes for items set in bold that do not appear in the meal plans appear in chapter three.

A WEEK'S MENUS—WOMEN

DAY ONE

BREAKFAST

Orange-Banana-Strawberry Soy Protein Shake *(orange/yellow; red/purple)* (see recipe on page 48)

LUNCH

Chicken Breast Seven Color Salad *(all colors)* (see recipe on page 48)

SNACK

½ medium cantaloupe *(orange)*

DINNER

Shrimp, Tofu, and Broccoli Stir-Fry *(green; white/green)* (see recipe on page 49)
½ cup steamed brown rice

SNACK

1 large nectarine *(orange/yellow)*

DAY TWO

BREAKFAST

Soy Nugget Cereal with Fruit
½ cup soy nugget cereal
1 cup nonfat milk
1 cup fresh blueberries *(red/purple)*

LUNCH

Tuna Niçoise Salad *(yellow/green; red; orange/yellow)* (see recipe on page 51)

SNACK

1 Fresh Orange *(orange/yellow)*

DINNER

Tomato-Soy Bisque *(white/green; orange; red)* (see recipe page 52)
Pan-Seared Cod with Balsamic Vinegar and Thyme (see recipe on page 53)
Sautéed Swiss Chard *(green)* (see recipe page on 54)
Whole-Wheat Couscous
  ½ cup cooked according to package directions

SNACK

½ fresh mango with lime juice *(orange)*

DAY THREE

BREAKFAST

Oatmeal and Eggs
  1 cup cooked oatmeal, made with 1 cup soy milk and sprin-
    kled with cinnamon
  4 egg whites, scrambled with onion, chives, and fresh herbs
    (white/green)

⅔ cup fresh orange juice *(orange/yellow)*

LUNCH

Open-Face Turkey/Avocado Sandwich
  1 slice whole-grain bread
  3 ounces roasted turkey breast
  ¼ fresh avocado *(yellow/green)*
  1 sliced tomato *(red)*
  Dijon-style mustard

Chopped Vegetable Salad *(all colors)* (see recipe page 54)

SNACK

1 cup fresh blackberries *(red/purple)*

DINNER

Whole-Wheat Pasta with Soy Meat Sauce *(red; white/green; orange; yellow/green)* (see recipe on page 56)

Green Salad
Mixed field greens with lemon-and-garlic dressing *(yellow/green)*

SNACK

1 cup cantaloupe balls sprinkled with fresh mint *(orange)*

DAY FOUR

BREAKFAST

½ toasted whole-grain English muffin, topped with ¾ cup nonfat
   cottage cheese and sprinkled with cinnamon
3 slices soy Canadian bacon
1 cup diced pineapple *(orange/yellow)*

LUNCH

Veggie burger on a whole-grain bun
Cabbage and Bell Pepper Slaw *(green; yellow/green)* (see recipe on
   page 57)

SNACK

1½ cups fresh strawberries *(red/purple)*

DINNER

Halibut and Vegetable Kabobs *(yellow/green; red; white/green)*
   (see recipe on page 59)
Cracked-wheat pilaf
Fresh baby carrots steamed with rice vinegar and fresh dill *(orange)*

SNACK

1 medium red pear poached with nutmeg and cloves *(red/purple)*

DAY FIVE

BREAKFAST

Breakfast Burritos *(red; yellow/green; white/green)* (see recipe on page
   60)
½ large papaya with lime juice *(orange/yellow)*

LUNCH

Chicken and Brown Rice Bowl *(green; orange; white/green)* (see recipe on page 61)

SNACK

1½ cups mixed berries *(red/purple)*

DINNER

Spicy Fish Stew *(red; yellow/green; white/green)* (see recipe on page 63)
Tossed green salad *(yellow/green)*

SNACK

1 large kiwi, diced and served with a handful of raspberries *(yellow/green)*

DAY SIX

BREAKFAST

Egg White Omelet with Spinach, Onion, Mushrooms, Tomatoes, and Mixed Herbs *(white/green; yellow/green; red)* (see recipe on page 64)
1 slice whole-grain bread
½ medium cantaloupe *(orange/yellow)*

LUNCH

Pita Pocket Tuna Sandwich *(orange; yellow/green; red)* (see recipe on page 65)
1 cup mixed vegetable juice *(red)*

SNACK

1 small banana

DINNER

Sweet-and-Sour Stuffed Cabbage *(green; red; white/green)* (see recipe on page 66)
Marinated Cucumber Salad *(white/green)* (see recipe on page 68)
4 ounce glass red wine *(red/purple)*

DAY SEVEN

BREAKFAST

Fresh Fruit and Yogurt Sundae
> Fruit salad of berries, peaches, and pineapple (red/purple, orange/yellow) on top of 1 cup plain yogurt, sprinkled with cinnamon, a drizzle of honey, and soy cereal for crunch.

1 slice whole-grain toast

LUNCH

Chef's Salad with Balsamic Vinaigrette *(yellow/green; red)* (see recipe on page 69)
3 whole-grain rye crackers

SNACK

Soy Protein Shake
> 1 cup soy milk
> ½ frozen banana
> 2 teaspoons honey
> Handful of frozen strawberries *(red/purple)*

Mix together in a blender.

DINNER

Barbecue Dinner
> 3-ounce chicken breast grilled with barbecue sauce
> 1 ear yellow corn, steamed or grilled *(yellow/green)*
> 2 cups steamed broccoli, spinach, and carrots seasoned with lemon and garlic *(green, yellow/green, orange, white/green)*

1 cup cubed watermelon *(red)*

A WEEK'S MENUS—MEN

DAY ONE

BREAKFAST

Orange-Banana-Strawberry Soy Protein Shake *(orange/yellow; red/purple)* (see recipe on page 48)
1 slice whole-grain toast

LUNCH

Chicken Breast Seven Color Salad *(all colors)* (see recipe on page 48)

SNACK

Quick Pizza Snack
    1 toasted whole-grain English muffin topped with:
    Prepared pizza sauce
    Few slices soy bacon or ham
    Shredded nonfat mozzarella cheese

Broil until hot.

DINNER

Shrimp, Tofu, and Broccoli Stir-Fry *(green, white/green)* (see recipe on page 49)
1 cup steamed brown rice

SNACK

Fruit Bowl
    1 large nectarine, diced *(orange/yellow)*
    ½ medium cantaloupe, diced *(orange)*
    Fresh mint, for sprinkling

DAY TWO

BREAKFAST

Soy Nugget Cereal with Fruit
    ½ cup soy nugget cereal
    1 cup nonfat milk
    1 cup fresh blueberries *(red/purple)*

LUNCH

Tuna Niçoise Salad *(yellow/green; red; orange/yellow)* (see recipe on page 51)

1 whole-wheat french roll

SNACK

Soy Smoothie

    1 scoop soy protein powder
    ½ cup orange juice
    ½ cup cold water
    A few ice cubes

Mix all ingredients in a blender.

DINNER

Tomato-Soy Bisque *(white/green; orange; red)* (see recipe on page 52)

Pan-Seared Cod with Balsamic Vinegar and Thyme (see recipe on page 53)

Sautéed Swiss Chard *(green)* (see recipe on page 54)

1 cup whole-wheat couscous

SNACK

½ fresh mango with lime juice *(orange)*

DAY THREE

BREAKFAST

Oatmeal and Eggs

    1½ cups cooked oatmeal, made with soy milk and sprinkled with cinnamon
    6 egg whites, scrambled with onion, chives, and fresh herbs *(white/green)*

⅔ cup fresh orange juice *(orange/yellow)*

LUNCH

Turkey/Avocado Sandwich
  2 slices whole-grain bread
  6 ounces roasted turkey breast
  ½ fresh avocado *(yellow/green)*
  1 sliced tomato *(red)*
  Dijon-style mustard

Chopped Vegetable Salad *(all colors)*(see recipe on page 54)

SNACK

Quick Tofu Fruit Pudding
  4 ounces soft tofu
  1 cup mixed berries (fresh or frozen) *(red/purple)*
  2 tablespoons orange juice concentrate
  2 to 3 teaspoons honey

Mix in a blender.

DINNER

Whole-Wheat Pasta with Soy Meat Sauce *(red; white/green;orange; yellow/green)* (see recipe on page 56)
Green Salad
  Mixed field greens with lemon-and-garlic dressing *(yellow/green)*

SNACK

1 cup cantaloupe balls sprinkled with fresh mint *(orange)*

DAY FOUR

BREAKFAST

1 toasted whole-grain English muffin, topped with 1 cup nonfat
  cottage cheese and sprinkled with cinnamon
3 slices soy Canadian bacon
1 cup fresh blackberries and raspberries *(red/purple)*

LUNCH

Veggie burger on a whole-grain bun

Cabbage and Bell Pepper Slaw *(green; yellow/green)* (see recipe on page 57)

SNACK

Hawaiian Smoothie

½ cup *each* pineapple juice and crushed pineapple *(orange/yellow)*

1 tablespoon apricot jam

½ banana

6 ounces lite firm tofu

Mix in a blender.

DINNER

Halibut and Vegetable Kabobs *(yellow/green; red; white/green)* (see recipe on page 59)

Cracked-wheat pilaf

Fresh baby carrots steamed with rice vinegar and fresh dill *(orange)*

SNACK

1 medium red pear poached with nutmeg and cloves *(red/purple)*

DAY FIVE

BREAKFAST

Breakfast Burrito *(yellow/green; red; white/green)* (see recipe on page 60)

½ large papaya with lime juice *(orange/yellow)*

LUNCH

Chicken and Brown Rice Bowl *(green; orange; white/green)* (see recipe on page 61)

SNACK

> ½ cup soy cereal
> 1 cup nonfat milk
> 1 cup mixed berries *(red/purple)*

DINNER

Spicy Fish Stew *(red; yellow/green; white/green)* (see recipe on page 63)
Tossed green salad *(yellow/green)*
1 whole-grain sourdough roll

SNACK

1 large kiwi, diced and served with a handful of raspberries *(yellow/ green)*

DAY SIX

BREAKFAST

Egg White Omelet with Spinach, Onions, Mushrooms, Tomatoes, and Mixed Herbs *(red; white/green; yellow/green)* (see recipe on page 64)
2 slices whole-grain bread
½ medium cantaloupe *(orange/yellow)*

LUNCH

Pita Pocket Tuna Sandwich *(orange; yellow/green; red)* (see recipe on page 65)
1 cup mixed vegetable juice *(red)*

SNACK

1 cup prepared vegetarian chili with 2 to 4 whole-grain crackers

DINNER

Sweet-and-Sour Stuffed Cabbage *(green; red; white/green)* (see recipe on page 66)
Marinated Cucumber Salad *(white/green)* (see recipe on page 68)
4 ounces red wine *(red/purple)*

DAY SEVEN

BREAKFAST

Fresh Fruit and Yogurt Sundae
   Fruit salad of berries, peaches, and pineapple *(red/purple, orange/yellow)* on top of 1 cup plain yogurt, sprinkled with cinnamon, a drizzle of honey, and soy cereal for crunch.
2 slices whole-grain toast

LUNCH

Chef's Salad with Balsamic Vinaigrette *(yellow/green; red)* (see recipe on page 69)
6 whole-grain crackers

SNACK

Soy Protein Shake
   1 cup soy milk
   1 frozen banana
   2 teaspoons honey
   Handful of frozen strawberries *(red/purple)*

Mix in a blender.

DINNER

Barbecue Dinner
   6 ounces chicken breast grilled with barbecue sauce
   2 ears yellow corn, steamed or grilled *(yellow/green)*
   2 cups steamed broccoli, spinach and carrots with lemon and garlic *(green, yellow/green, orange, white/green)*
1 cup cubed watermelon *(red)*

Now that you have seen what a week's worth of menus looks like, you can customize your own meals by using the charts that follow. This will help you choose the foods you love, which may or may not be in the sample meals shown. You will see that for each type of food, there is a serving size with an approximate calorie content. There is a table for the seven fruit and vegetable color groups, a table for proteins, one for grains, and one for taste enhancers/calorie boosters.

If you are female, choose the following each day:

❖ One serving of each of the seven color-coded groups of fruits or vegetables

❖ 3 to 4 units of protein (half animal protein, half soy)

❖ 3 to 4 whole-grain servings

❖ 2 to 3 taste enhancers

If you are male, choose the following each day:

❖ One serving of each of the seven color-coded fruits and vegetables

❖ 7 to 9 units of protein (half animal protein, half soy)

❖ 5 to 6 whole-grain servings

❖ 4 to 5 taste enhancers

You can adjust the servings up or down depending on your calorie needs, but these are the portions that were used to plan the week's menus. You can also use these tables to make substitutions on the meal plans above by being careful to select servings with similar calorie levels from the tables.

PROTEINS

Women: 3 to 4 Units Per Day
Men: 7 to 9 Units Per Day

FOOD ITEM	ONE UNIT	CALORIES	PROTEIN (GM)
Chicken breast	3 ounces, cooked weight	140	25
Cod	3 ounces, cooked weight	90	19
Crab	4 ounces, cooked weight	110	22
Egg whites	6 whites	100	21
Flounder, sole	3 ounces, cooked weight	100	20
Halibut	3 ounces, cooked weight	120	23
Lobster	4 ounces, cooked weight	110	23
Nonfat cottage cheese	¾ cup	105	21
Nonfat milk + egg white	1 cup milk + 4 egg whites	150	22
Nonfat milk	1 cup	90	9
Plain yogurt	1 cup	135	14
Salmon	3 ounces, cooked weight	155	21
Scallops	3 ounces, cooked weight	100	19
Sea bass	3 ounces, cooked weight	105	20
Shrimp	4 ounces, cooked weight	110	24
Snapper	3 ounces, cooked weight	110	22
Soy milk + egg white	1 cup soy milk + 4 egg whites	150	21
Soy milk	1 cup	80	7
Swordfish	3 ounces, cooked weight	130	22
Tuna	3 ounces, water pack	110	20
Turkey breast	3 ounces, cooked weight	115	25

VEGETARIAN

FOOD ITEM	PORTION	CALORIES	PROTEIN (GM)
Soy burger or sausage	1 patty	100	18 (varies)
Soy Canadian bacon	3 slices	80	16 (varies)
Soy cereal	½ cup	140	25 (varies)
Soy ground round	½ cup	90	18

FOOD ITEM	PORTION	CALORIES	PROTEIN (GM)
Soy hot dog	2 links	110	22 (varies)
Soy protein powder	1 ounce	110	20
Tofu, firm	½ cup	180	20 (varies)

FRUITS AND VEGETABLES

Women and men:
Choose at least ONE item from each color group.

RED

FOOD ITEM	PORTION	CALORIES	FIBER
Pink grapefruit	1 whole fruit	75	3
Pink grapefruit juice	1 cup	95	0
Tomato juice	1 cup	40	1
Tomato sauce/puree	1 cup	100	5
Tomato soup, made with water	1 cup	85	0
Tomato vegetable juice	1 cup	45	2
Tomatoes, cooked	1 cup	70	3
Tomatoes, raw	1 large	40	2
Watermelon	1 cup balls	50	1

RED/PURPLE

FOOD ITEM	PORTION	CALORIES	FIBER
Beets, cooked	1 cup	75	3
Blackberries	1 cup	75	8
Blueberries	1 cup	110	5
Cherries	1 cup	85	3
Cranberries	1 cup raw	60	5
Cranberry juice	⅔ cup	100	0
Cranberry sauce	¼ cup	100	1
Eggplant, cooked	2 cups	60	5
Grape juice	⅔ cup	100	0

FOOD ITEM	PORTION	CALORIES	FIBER
Grapes	1 cup	115	2
Peppers, red bell	1 large	45	3
Plums	3 small	100	3
Prunes	5 whole	100	3
Red apple	1 medium	100	4
Red cabbage, cooked	2 cups	60	6
Red pear	1 medium	100	4
Red wine	4 ounces	80	0
Strawberries	1 ½ cups, sliced	75	6

ORANGE

FOOD ITEM	PORTION	CALORIES	FIBER
Acorn squash, baked	1 cup	85	6
Apricot	5 whole	85	4
Cantaloupe	½ medium	80	2
Carrot juice	1 cup	95	2
Carrots, cooked	1 cup	70	5
Carrots, raw	3 medium	75	6
Mango	½ large	80	3
Pumpkin, cooked	1 cup	50	3
Sweet potato	1 small, 2" × 5"	100	2
Winter squash, baked	1 cup	70	7

ORANGE/YELLOW

FOOD ITEM	PORTION	CALORIES	FIBER
Nectarine	1 large	70	2
Orange	1 large	85	4
Orange juice	⅔ cup	75	0
Papaya	½ large	75	3
Peach	1 large	70	3
Peach nectar	⅔ cup	90	1
Pineapple	1 cup, diced	75	2
Tangerine	2 medium	85	5
Tangerine juice	⅔ cup	75	0
Yellow grapefruit	1 fruit	75	2

YELLOW/GREEN

FOOD ITEM	PORTION	CALORIES	FIBER
Avocado	½ average fruit	80	2
Collard greens, cooked	2 cups	100	10
Corn	½ cup kernels or 1 ear	75	2
Cucumber	1 average	40	2
Green beans, cooked	2 cups	85	8
Green peas	½ cup	70	4
Green bell peppers	1 large	45	3
Honeydew	¼ large melon	100	2
Kiwi	1 large	55	3
Mustard greens, cooked	2 cups	40	6
Romaine lettuce	4 cups	30	4
Spinach, cooked	2 cups	80	8
Spinach, raw	4 cups	30	4
Turnip greens, cooked	2 cups	60	10
Yellow bell peppers	1 large	50	2
Zucchini with skin, cooked	2 cups	60	5

GREEN

FOOD ITEM	PORTION	CALORIES	FIBER
Broccoli, cooked	2 cups	85	9
Brussels sprouts, cooked	1 cup	60	4
Cabbage, cooked	2 cups	70	8
Cabbage, raw	2 cups	40	4
Cauliflower, cooked	2 cups	55	6
Chinese cabbage, cooked	2 cups	40	5
Kale, cooked	2 cups	70	5
Swiss chard, cooked	2 cups	70	7

WHITE/GREEN

FOOD ITEM	PORTION	CALORIES	FIBER
Artichoke	1 medium	60	6
Asparagus	18 spears	60	4
Celery	3 large stalks	30	3

FOOD ITEM	PORTION	CALORIES	FIBER
Chives	2 tablespoons	2	0
Endive, raw	½ head	45	8
Garlic	1 clove	5	0
Leeks, cooked	1 medium	40	1
Mushrooms, cooked	1 cup	40	3
Onion	1 large	60	3

GRAINS

Women: 3 to 4 Portions Per Day
Men: 5 to 6 Portions Per Day

FOOD ITEM	PORTION	CALORIES	FIBER
100% bran	½ cup	90	10
40% bran	½ cup	80	3
Barley	½ cup, cooked	95	3
Bran flakes	¾ cup	100	5
Brown rice	½ cup, cooked	110	2
Corn tortilla	2 medium	120	2
Couscous, whole wheat	½ cup, cooked	85	2
Cracked wheat	½ cup, cooked	75	4
Crackers, whole-rye wafers	1 triple cracker	85	5
English muffin, whole grain	1 whole	135	4
Oatmeal	⅔ cup, cooked	100	3
Puffed wheat	2 cups	100	3
Raisin bran	½ cup	90	2–4
Rye bread	1 slice	75	2
Shredded wheat	1 cup	110	3
Whole-grain bread	1 slice	70–100	2–4
Whole-grain hot cereal	½ cup, cooked	85	4
Whole-wheat pasta	½ cup, cooked	85	2
Wild rice	½ cup, cooked	80	1

TASTE ENHANCERS AND CALORIE BOOSTERS

Women: 2 to 3 Portions Per Day
Men: 4 to 5 Portions Per Day

FOOD ITEM	PORTION	CALORIES	FIBER	FAT (G)
Almonds	½ ounce (11 nuts)	85	2	7
Banana	1 small (6–7 inches)	90	2	0
Black beans	½ cup, cooked	115	7	0
Cashews, dry roasted	½ ounce	80	0	6
Cheese, mozzarella, part skim	1 ounce	80	0	5
Cheese, Parmesan	3 tablespoons	80	0	5
Cheese, reduced-fat cheddar	1 ounce	50	0	2
Garbanzo beans	½ cup, cooked	140	5	1
Kidney beans	½ cup, cooked	115	6	0
Lentils	½ cup, cooked	115	8	0
Macadamia nuts	½ ounce (5–6 nuts)	100	1	11
Olive oil	1 teaspoon	40	0	4
Olives	10 large	50	0	7
Peanuts, dry roasted	15 nuts	90	3	7
Pecans, dry roasted	½ ounce	95	1	9
Pignola (pine nuts)	1 tablespoon (40 nuts)	50	1	4
Pinto beans	½ cup, cooked	115	7	0
Pistachios, dry roasted	½ ounce	85	2	7
Potato, baked	½ large	110	2	0
Sesame seeds	1 tablespoon	50	2	7
Split peas	½ cup, cooked	115	8	0
Sunflower seed kernels	½ ounce	80	2	7
Walnuts	½ ounce (7 halves)	90	3	9

Now you have a good idea of how the Color Code looks and how you can put it into effect. Remember, while this is not a weight-loss diet, many people lose some weight as they substitute the healthy foods above for some of the high-fat/high-sugar snacks—the cakes, pastries, and chips—they usually eat.

As you start to implement this diet, the next few chapters will give you more practical hints on how to fit the Color Code into your busy lifestyle.

3

Using the Color Code

You are about to start using the Color Code, but what do you do first? This chapter is all about getting your house in order, starting with your kitchen. I decided to start with your kitchen because that is where you will eat in those unplanned moments at night and on weekends. It's where you sometimes start your day off on the wrong foot, and end your day drowning in the wrong snack foods. I recognize that you probably eat a lot of your food on the run, in restaurants, in your car, and in airports. The chapter that follows this one is all about traveling and dining with the Color Code. If you absolutely never eat at home, skip ahead. Otherwise, get ready to stock your pantry and master your market shopping routine.

If You Don't Buy It, You Can't Eat It

There's an old saying that if you don't buy something and you don't put it in your pantry or refrigerator, you can't eat it. So go through your kitchen and get rid of those foods that modern advertising has empowered with the ability to reduce your stress, make you strong, wake you up when you're tired, or make you happy. Food cannot give you a good time, only you can do that. What snack foods do is trade an overstated taste of salty, sweet, or fatty for a momentary pleasure followed by weight gain. Not only do you feel less happy being overweight, but your health suffers as these snack foods replace the healthy fruits and vegetables you should be eating instead. By replacing snack foods with healthy fruits and vegetables you will be putting into your kitchen a garden food pharmacy with the power to protect your DNA and help prevent a number of common diseases.

The Clean Sweep

At least at the beginning, and until you retrain your taste buds, remove all the weakest foods, those with little color, from your pantry and refrigerator. As you will read later on, these are the foods that cause an imbalance in your DNA and turn your normal protective reactions against you. Start with the bottom of the USDA pyramid and remove all refined carbohydrates, including pasta, rice, low-fiber cereals, pancake and cookie mixes, white breads, and bagels, and put them aside. If you can't bring yourself to throw them away, put some in freezer bags and store them so they won't be as available. You will want to replace these with high-fiber breads and whole grains. As a routine, I freeze even high-fiber breads so they are eaten more slowly and you don't end up throwing away moldy breads on a regular basis. By cleaning out the bottom of the pyramid until it contains only whole-grain, high-fiber foods, you will be attacking one of the primary sources of excess calories for most Americans, which accounts for the run of so-called low-"carb" diets. In fact, fruits and vegetables and whole grains are good "carbs" and will be the heart of your diet based on the Color Code.

Trimming Away Excess Fat

Most foods have some fat, but you can balance the fat in your diet to better reflect what your body has evolved to expect by taking the following steps. First, get rid of margarines, mayonnaise, vegetable shortenings, and vegetable oils, including safflower, sunflower, cottonseed, and corn oils. These oils are loaded with up to 60 or 70 percent of omega-6 polyunsaturated fats, which promote DNA damage. If you have canola oil or olive oil, keep those; they are used strategically to increase taste as needed in our recipes.

Next, give away or throw away your whole milk and cheeses. Those high-fat, calorie-loaded cheese slices provide between 80 and 140 calories per one-ounce slice, depending on the fat content. You can replace whole milk with nonfat, lactase-treated milk, or, even better, a soy milk. Much of the world's population cannot digest milk efficiently. With 40 percent of our population suffering gastrointestinal upset after drinking milk, maybe this is an area you should examine. The latest dietary guidelines from the USDA finally recognize soy milk for protein as an alternative to cow's milk. Calcium is another matter we will discuss later.

You cannot go on a zero-fat diet. Even fruits and vegetables have some fat, but they are balanced between the omega-3 and omega-6 varieties, as well as the healthy monounsaturated fatty acids found in olive oil. When these healthy elements were stripped out of vegetable oils, our bodies became overloaded with the wrong types of fats. By taking in more omega-3 fats that exist naturally in foods, with fewer added omega-6 fats, you are just correcting the balance in your kitchen.

Redesigning Your Dinner Plate

The size and contents of your dinner plate are important. The average restaurant plate has increased in size from a ten-inch diameter to a fourteen-inch diameter. At home you want to use standard plates and imagine portion sizes that are much smaller than what you eat in the restaurant. It is easy to visualize your plate (see page 46) as containing meats, starchy vegetables, and little or no colorful vegetables.

The typical American restaurant plate has nine to fourteen ounces of red meat, mashed potatoes, and corn. With the exception of the yellow in corn, the meal provides little in the way of colorful chemicals.

To change your plate, first reduce your meat portion to three to six ounces and switch from mashed potatoes to sliced carrots, and from corn to spinach.

Then, as you refine your color code, add more colors to your plate with few extra calories. Add red pepper, tomato sauce, garlic or onions,

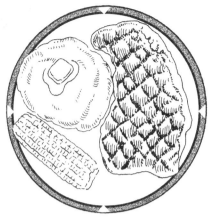

Step 1:
Starting point for a
typical American plate

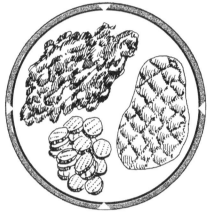

Step 2:
Toward a healthier plate

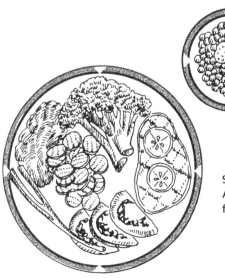

Step 3:
A healthy colorful plate with
fruit/berry dessert

broccoli, and the rinds of oranges or lemons to top off your chicken or fish. Add a mixed berries dessert for red/purple foods.

So, now you have less fat, more phytochemicals, and fewer calories.

The Heart of the Colorful Kitchen: Fruits and Vegetables

If you look around your kitchen, your fruits and vegetables probably reflect the poor variety found in most U.S. households. If your kitchen contains mostly bananas and apples, you need to make some changes. You can easily fill your kitchen with a rainbow selection of the right fruits and vegetables in great variety and at a low cost.

First of all, you have lots of good choices in your local grocery store, but they are not all in the produce section. Fresh fruits and vegetables are great, but they are only one choice. Frozen fruits and vegetables are picked fresh and at a just-ripe stage to maximize their taste. Fresh fruits and vegetables have to be picked while they can still withstand the long trip to your local market. The best example of this is the tomato, which is picked while still green and sprayed with gas to stimulate the development of red color. Apples can be stored for many months under nitrogen gas before they make the trip to the market.

Seasonal fruits and vegetables are more varied and are affordable, except when they are out of season. If you don't mind the taste of frozen fruits and vegetables, you can enjoy strawberries, raspberries, blueberries, spinach, broccoli, and many other fruits and vegetables year-round no matter where you live. When it comes to tomatoes, heat processing releases the red pigment, lycopene, so it can be absorbed into your body. So stock up on tomato sauces, tomato soups, and tomato and mixed-vegetable juices. As little as six ounces of mixed-vegetable juice can significantly increase the levels of lycopene in your body, where it is able to act to protect your DNA. Since boiling removes some of the water-soluble chemicals and vitamins from vegetables, I recommend that you steam vegetables by using a double boiler or a metal colander in a pot with a little water in the bottom. You can also steam vegetables in microwave-safe dishes in the microwave, in bamboo containers, or in appliances designed just for the purpose of steaming vegetables. If your market has a salad bar, you can often find a variety of items for a colorful salad, or prewashed-and-cut vegetables that can be quickly steamed for a healthy side dish.

Color Code Foods Made Easy

Here is a breakdown by Color Code of the most convenient ways to get your fruits and veggies:

Red group: canned or bottled tomato juice and mixed vegetable juice; canned tomatoes, tomato paste, tomato sauce, pasta sauces; prepared tomato soup; prepared tomato salsa; chilled, presliced pink grapefruit; precut watermelon in season

Red/purple group: Bottled grape juice (100 percent juice), bottled cranberry juice or frozen cranberry juice concentrate, frozen whole berries, preshredded purple cabbage for cooking or slaws, frozen sliced peppers, and fresh apples, pears, berries, and cherries.

Orange group: Prewashed and cut or shredded carrots, frozen carrots, and frozen winter squash; presliced mango available fresh-chilled or packed in juice or as frozen mango chunks; precut cantaloupe wedges or balls; and whole fresh apricots.

Orange/yellow group: Fresh orange juice, frozen orange juice or tangerine juice concentrate; presliced papaya, pineapple, and yellow grapefruit sections available fresh or chilled and packed in juice; frozen pineapple chunks; pineapple canned in pineapple juice; fresh whole nectarines, oranges, peaches, and tangerines.

Yellow/green group: Fresh or frozen spinach, collard greens, mustard greens, avocados, and turnip greens. Loose-pack spinach in bags is particularly convenient because you can add only what you need to soups, mixed dishes, omelets, and pasta. Frozen pepper slices are easily added to dishes, and prewashed salad greens and raw spinach make quick work of a colorful salad. Look, too, for precut honeydew melon.

Green group: Prewashed-and-cut broccoli florets and broccoli stems for slaw, and broccoli sprouts, make getting these healthy vegetables much easier. Preshredded cabbage for cooking or for slaw, prewashed-and-cut cauliflower florets, and frozen broccoli and cauliflower are also widely available.

White/green group: If you don't like preparing onions and garlic, you can find prechopped garlic in jars and packaged, prechopped fresh onion in the produce section. Washed and sliced celery stalks are great for snacking, and sliced mushrooms are available packaged and at many supermarket salad bars.

Spices and Other Staples

When you are stocking up on staples, don't forget to get some spices. Spices, nuts, seeds, and oils are all taste enhancers. This is especially true with steamed vegetables, which often have subtle, mild tastes or mildly unpleasant tastes that need dressing up. Spices can be used to contrast two flavors. For example, ginger and garlic are contrasting and can be used with cut-up broccoli or Brussels sprouts. Rosemary, oregano, or thyme can be used with carrots, and dill, which is famous with fish dishes, can also be used with summer squash or zucchini. Be imaginative—try some new spice combinations.

Salsa and chili peppers can add excitement to any vegetable dish, and they contain a chemical called "capsaicin," which has been shown to have anticancer effects. Citrus fruits including tangerines, oranges, and lemons can also be mixed with these dishes, and you can use small amounts of olive or canola oils or pan sprays for sautéeing dishes or for wok cooking. Remember, you are not trying to eliminate all fat and refined carbohydrates, just the excess amounts used to hook you into buying certain types of foods. Use small amounts to make your food taste great. You'll find it doesn't take much, and after a few weeks of eating lower-fat foods, you won't be able to stand the high-fat foods served in most coffee shops and restaurants.

Super Soy Protein Solutions

A great staple for your cupboard is isolated soy protein powder. This can be added to many different dishes to fortify them with high-quality protein without affecting the taste. You can add soy protein powder to pasta sauces and to fruit juices. The low-fat diets of the early 1980s often did not include enough protein. Soy protein powder taken as a shake or added to various dishes can reduce your hunger between meals and helps to maintain your muscle protein by providing high-quality protein.

Introducing soy protein into your diet is made easier with convenient soy protein meat substitutes that are precooked and are available fresh, frozen, and, occasionally, dehydrated. Soy "ground round" works especially well in dishes calling for ground meat. Tofu, available fresh (water-packed) or aseptically packaged (on the shelf), can be mashed, diced, pureed, frozen, and crumbled, and takes on the flavor of the dishes to which it is added.

Cold cereals with soy in them are another easy way to boost your soy intake. Many cold cereals make great snack foods straight from the box. If you prefer hot cereals, quick-cooking rolled oats and instant oatmeal and whole-grain hot cereals in single-serving packets or plastic containers are great for breakfast and snacks.

Quick-cooking brown rice and soba (buckwheat) noodles can be the basis for a quick meal with precut vegetables and boneless, skinless poultry breast or fish. Cracked wheat cooks quickly and can be used as a side dish or as a basis for a salad; and whole-wheat couscous, which practically cooks itself, makes a delicious high-fiber side dish. Look for high-fiber whole grain (100 percent whole-wheat flour as the first ingredient) in breads, crackers, and flat breads for "wraps."

Sometimes You Feel Like a Nut

Almonds, walnuts, pistachios, and macadamia nuts are wonderful staples that can enhance your cooking, but don't break into your cupboard to eat the whole can. You only need a few nuts to get the amount of monounsaturated fat your body needs and to enhance taste. Try toasting nuts in a toaster or in a pan with a spray of olive oil to bring out their flavor. You can also use almond slivers, which give a great taste dividend without a lot of extra calories. A handful of nuts is about 100 calories, so use them cautiously and, unless you are planning a long hike in the mountains, don't eat a large bowl of peanuts.

Filling Up with Air-Popped Popcorn

If you want a food to eat while watching television, your best bet is air-popped popcorn made in an air popper. An air popper usually costs under twenty dollars and works by blowing hot air over popcorn kernels, which naturally contain water. As the water is heated within the hard shell of the popcorn kernel, it finally breaks the shell, making popcorn. You don't need any cooking oil or spray to make air-popped popcorn. Eat it while it is still steaming and you have a tasty dish—and your fingers won't be greasy, which is a real break for your couch. A ten-pound bag of plain popcorn kernels is a great staple to have on hand.

Use these recipes for inspiration, and experiment with new vegetables and seasonings that please your own taste buds. If you have farmers' markets nearby, you should seek out the freshest fruits and vegetables in season, and you might be exposed to new foods you haven't tried. If an ingredient appeals to you, use it as an addition or replacement food in the recipe. Cooking is meant to be a creative experience, not a chore, so do experiment. All these recipes were designed to maximize the health-giving properties of colorful fruits and vegetables, with a minimum of fat, a reasonable number of calories, and an abundance of flavor.

Color Code Recipes

Orange-Banana-Strawberry
  Soy Protein Shake
Chicken Breast Seven
  Color Salad
Shrimp, Tofu and
  Broccoli Stir-Fry
Tuna Niçoise Salad
Tomato-Soy Bisque
Pan-Seared Cod with Balsamic
  Vinegar and Thyme
Sautéed Swiss Chard
Chopped Vegetable Salad
Soy Meat Sauce for Pasta

Cabbage and Bell Pepper Slaw
Halibut and Vegetable Kabobs
Breakfast Burritos
Chicken and Brown Rice Bowl
Spicy Fish Stew
Egg White Omelet with Spinach,
   Onion, Mushrooms, Tomatoes,
   and Mixed Herbs
Pita Pocket Tuna Sandwich
Sweet-and-Sour Stuffed Cabbage
Marinated Cucumber Salad
Chef's Salad with Balsamic
   Vinaigrette

Orange-Banana-Strawberry Soy Protein Shake

(orange/yellow; red/purple)

Soy protein shakes can be made with virtually any juices and fruits. This version is one of our favorites. If you use frozen fruit, the shake will be very thick; if you use fresh berries, you can add a few ice cubes if you want.
SERVES 1.

> 1 ounce plain or vanilla-flavored soy protein isolate powder
>   (or amount to supply approximately 20 grams of protein)
> ½ cup water
> ½ cup orange juice *(orange/yellow)*
> 1½ cups fresh or frozen strawberries *(red/purple)*
> ½ banana

Place all ingredients in the blender and blend until smooth.

NUTRITIONAL ANALYSIS PER SERVING: Calories: 282 • Protein: 25 grams • Fat: 2 grams • Carbohydrate: 49 grams • Fiber: 8 grams • α-carotene: 16 μg; • β-carotene: 42 μg • β-cryptoxantin 123 μg • lutein + zeaxanthin: 171 μg

Chicken Breast Seven Color Salad

This colorful salad goes together very quickly if you have cooked chicken breasts on hand. Preparing extra chicken breasts is always a good idea, since they can be frozen and then thawed out whenever needed. All the color groups are represented in this salad, and the dressing complements the ingredients beautifully. SERVES 1.

> SALAD:
> 2 chicken breast halves, marinated in teriyaki sauce, grilled,
>   refrigerated
> 1 pear, peeled and cubed
> 10 red grapes (red/purple)
> 1 small can mandarin oranges, drained (yellow/orange)
> 1 yellow pepper, sliced julienne (yellow/green)
> 1 carrot, julienne sliced (orange)
> ¼ avocado, cubed (yellow/green)

2 green onions, chopped (white/green)
10 cherry tomatoes (red)
1 cup broccoli florets (green)
1 package european lettuce mix or raw spinach

DRESSING:
1 tablespoon rice vinegar
2 teaspoons soy sauce
½ teaspoon sugar
1/8 teaspoon powdered ginger
¼ teaspoon sesame oil
⅛ teaspoon white pepper

Slice grilled chicken breasts into strips and place in large salad bowl with other salad ingredients. In a small bowl, whisk together dressing ingredients. Pour dressing over salad and toss.

NUTRITIONAL ANALYSIS PER SERVING: Calories: 328 • Protein: 32 grams • Fat: 5 grams • Carbohydrate: 42 grams • Fiber: 10 grams • α-carotene: 689 μg; • β-carotene: 2524 μg • β-cryptoxanthin 204 μg • lutein + zeaxanthin: 1392 μg

Shrimp, Tofu, and Broccoli Stir-Fry *(green; white/green)*

Stir-frying is one of the healthiest ways to prepare foods if you use a minimum amount of oil. Foods are cut into bite-size pieces so they cook quickly, and are cooked only until crisp-tender, which retains nutrients. This beautiful combination of shrimp and bright green broccoli is protein-enriched with tofu, and features a tangy ginger-and-garlic sauce enhanced with a surprise ingredient—a touch of ketchup. SERVES 2

12 ounces raw shrimp, fresh or frozen, shelled and deveined
4 cups fresh broccoli florets *(green)*
Nonstick pan spray
1 clove garlic, minced *(white/green)*
¼ inch-thick slice fresh gingerroot, peeled and finely minced
1 scallion, minced *(white/green)*
4 ounces firm tofu, cubed into ½ inch dice

SAUCE INGREDIENTS

2 tablespoons low-sodium soy sauce

3 tablespoons rice wine or chicken broth

2 teaspoons rice vinegar

½ teaspoon sugar

1 tablespoon prepared ketchup *(red)*

⅛ teaspoon ground white pepper

3 teaspoons cornstarch

If shrimp is frozen, defrost according to package directions. Blanch broccoli florets by dropping into boiling water for 1 minute. Drain, but do not rinse, cover and set aside. Combine sauce ingredients in a small saucepan over medium-high heat and cook, stirring, until mixture boils, thickens and clears. Set sauce aside.

Spray a large skillet with pan spray. Heat skillet over high heat. When hot, add garlic, ginger, and scallions. Stir-fry for a few seconds, but do not allow the garlic to brown. Add the shrimp and continue to stir-fry until the shrimp is pink and almost cooked through. Add the tofu and blanched broccoli florets and stir-fry for another two minutes, until the tofu is hot. Finally, pour in the sauce mixture and stir quickly to mix. Serve over steamed brown rice.

NUTRITIONAL ANALYSIS PER SERVING: Calories: 358 • Protein: 50 grams • Fat: 8 grams • Carbohydrate: 23 grams • Fiber: 6 grams • β-carotene: 1471 µg • lutein + zeaxanthin: 4303 µg; lycopene: 1276 µg

Tuna Niçoise Salad *(yellow/green; red; orange/yellow)*

A true Niçoise salad always contains tuna, potatoes, and green beans, and never vinegar in the dressing. This version gets additional color from the addition of tomato and deep green romaine lettuce. SERVES 2

> 4 cups romaine lettuce, torn into bite-size pieces *(yellow/ green)*
>
> 6 ounces water-packed tuna, flaked
>
> 2 cups French-cut green beans, steamed until crisp-tender, then chilled *(yellow/green)*
>
> 1 fresh tomato, diced *(red)*
>
> 2 small red new potatoes, boiled until tender, chilled and sliced
>
> DRESSING:
>
> 2 tablespoons olive oil
>
> 1 tablespoon fresh lemon juice *(orange/yellow)*
>
> ¼ teaspoon sugar
>
> ¼ teaspoon dried dill *or* 1 teaspoon fresh
>
> ¼ teaspoon salt
>
> Freshly ground pepper to taste
>
> ½ teaspoon Dijon-style mustard

Whisk dressing ingredients in a small bowl or shake together in a jar and set aside. Divide romaine leaves onto two plates. Arrange the tuna, beans, tomatoes, olives, and pototoes on top of the romaine. Drizzle the dressing over the tuna and vegetables.

NUTRITIONAL ANALYSIS PER SERVING: Calories: 306 • Protein: 29 grams • Fat: 7 grams • Carbohydrate: 34 grams • Fiber: 9 grams • α-carotene: 186 μg; • β-carotene: 2246 μg • lutein + zeaxanthin: 3862 μg • lycopene: 2723 μg

Tomato-Soy Bisque *(white/green; orange; red)*

Unless you can find very ripe tomatoes, used canned plum tomatoes for tomato soup because they are more flavorful. The heat processing of canned tomatoes makes the beneficial lycopene in them more available to the body, too. The acidity in tomato soup is usually smoothed out with whole milk or cream, but in this bisque the tomatoes have been given a healthy protein bonus with soy milk. SERVES 8

> 1 tablespoon olive oil
> 2 medium onions, thinly sliced *(white/green)*
> 1 medium carrot, peeled and chopped *(orange)*
> 6 cloves garlic, coarsely chopped *(white/green)*
> 4 14½-ounce cans Italian plum tomatoes in their own juices
>   *(red)*
> 1 tablespoon fresh oregano leaves *or* 1 teaspoon dried
> Pinch of sugar
> Salt and freshly ground pepper to taste
> 4 cups low sodium chicken broth
> ½ teaspoon ground allspice
> 2 cups plain soy milk
> 1 teaspoon Worcestershire sauce

Heat the oil over medium heat in a large soup pot. Add the onions, carrot, and garlic, and cook until the vegetables have wilted, 8 to 10 minutes. Add the canned tomatoes with their juice, oregano, sugar, and salt and pepper. Cook for 5 minutes, breaking up the tomatoes. Add broth and allspice and slowly bring to a boil. Reduce the heat to low, partially cover, and simmer for 45 minutes. Puree the soup in batches in the blender. Return to the soup pot, stir in the soy milk and adjust seasonings, and heat through.

NUTRITIONAL ANALYSIS PER SERVING: Calories: 111 • Protein: 7 grams • Fat: 4 grams • Carbohydrate: 14 grams • Fiber: 4 grams • α-carotene: 291 µg; • β-carotene: 882 µg • lutein + zeaxanthin: 107 µg • lycopene: 19,959 µg

Pan-Seared Cod with Balsamic Vinegar and Thyme

This is one of the easiest ways to prepare fish. It comes out flaky, moist, and very flavorful and is a snap to make. This method can be adapted to any type of fish and can also be used for boneless, skinless chicken breasts. Fish should cook for about 10 minutes for each 1-inch thickness; chicken breast will need a total of about 15 minutes cooking time. SERVES 2

> 1 pound fresh cod filet
> Salt and freshly ground pepper to taste
> 2 teaspoons olive oil
> 2 tablespoons balsamic vinegar
> 1 tablespoon fresh thyme

Sprinkle fish with salt and freshly ground pepper on both sides. Heat a large skillet, for which you have a cover, over medium-high heat. When hot, add the olive oil. When the oil is hot, place the fish in the pan, lower the heat to medium and cook for 5 minutes, or until the underside is brown and a crust begins to form. Carefully turn the fish over, turn the heat down to medium low and cover the skillet. Cook for about five minutes more. Fish is done when it flakes with a fork. Remove fish from skillet and place on a plate. Bring the heat back up to medium high, add the balsamic vinegar and cook quickly, scraping the pan with a spatula. Turn off the heat, put the fish back in the skillet, and turn over to coat both sides with the reduced vinegar. Sprinkle with fresh thyme and serve immediately.

NUTRITIONAL ANALYSIS PER SERVING: Calories: 228 • Protein: 40 grams • Fat: 6 grams • Carbohydrate: 1 gram

Sautéed Swiss Chard *(green)*

Swiss chard tastes like "grown-up" spinach. The flavor is wonderful, and it is a nutrional powerhouse. You can commonly find white and red Swiss chard in the supermarket, but check your local farmers' markets for the newer varieties in purple, orange, and bright yellow. This simple method of cooking chard can also be used for spinach. SERVES 2

> 1 bunch fresh Swiss chard *(green)*
> 1½ teaspoons olive oil
> ¼ purple onion, very thinly sliced *(red/purple)*
> 2 cloves garlic, minced *(white/green)*
> Salt to taste

Wash the chard thoroughly and cut off the stems. Chop the leaves into large pieces and toss in a colander to dry the leaves. Heat a large skillet over medium-high heat, and add the olive oil. When the oil is hot, add the purple onion, and cook, stirring, just until onion softens. Add the chard and garlic, and cook and stir just until the chard wilts. Finally, add salt to taste, stir quickly, and serve immediately.

NUTRITIONAL ANALYSIS PER SERVING: Calories: 67 • Protein: 2.5 gm • Fat: 3 gm • Carbohydrate: 8 gm • Fiber: 2.5 gm • α-carotene: 55 μg; • β-carotene: 4389 μg

Chopped Vegetable Salad *(all colors)*

If there is one recipe that captures the Color Code, this is it. This is an absolutely beautiful salad with every color group represented. The contrast of the brightly colored vegetables and the black olives is eye-catching. Because the dressing contains fresh basil, which turns brown if it sits, this must be tossed just before serving. While it won't be as pretty the next day, it still tastes great. For the best display when freshly made, serve this in a white bowl. SERVES 8

> 1 bunch fresh broccoli *(green)*
> 1 small head fresh cauliflower *(green)*
> 2 cups raw baby carrots *(orange)*
> 1 basket cherry tomatoes, halved *(red)*

1 large cucumber, peeled and diced into large pieces
   (yellow/green)
1 red bell pepper, julienne cut *(red/purple)*
1 yellow bell pepper, julienne cut *(yellow/green)*
1 small purple onion, sliced paper thin *(red/purple)*
1 cup whole small black olives
¼ cup minced fresh parsley

DRESSING
2 tablespoons olive oil
1 tablespoon balsamic vinegar
2 tablespoons fresh lemon juice *(orange/yellow)*
½ cup fresh basil leaves
1 teaspoon salt
½ teaspoon freshly ground pepper
½ teaspon Dijon-style mustard
3 cloves garlic *(white/green)*

Bring a large pot of water to a boil. While waiting for the water to boil, break broccoli and cauliflower into small bite-size pieces. When water is boiling, add broccoli, cauliflower, and carrots, and cook for 2 minutes or until vegetables are slightly tender but still crisp. Drain and immediately rinse well with cold water to stop cooking. Place in refrigerator for 30 minutes to chill thoroughly.

Place all dressing ingredients in the blender and blend until basil and garlic are pureed. Dressing will be thick. Set aside.

In a large serving bowl, mix the blanched vegetables with the tomatoes, cucumber, peppers, onion, olives, and parsley. Add dressing and toss. Serve immediately.

NUTRITIONAL ANALYSIS PER SERVING: Calories: 90 • Protein: 5 grams • Fat: 2 grams • Carbohydrate: 4 grams • Fiber: 11 grams • α-carotene: 960 μg; • β-carotene: 1,954 μg • β-cryptoxantin: 136 μg • lutein + zeaxanthin: 440 μg • lycopene: 908 μg

Soy Meat Sauce for Pasta

One of the nice things about ground soy meat substitutes is that they readily take on the flavors of whatever they are cooked with. Since ground meats are often used in highly seasoned dishes such as chili, tacos, and pasta sauces, the soy substitute can often not be distinguised from meat. SERVES 4 GENEROUSLY

> 1 tablespoon olive oil
> 2 cloves garlic, minced *(white/green)*
> 1 medium onion, coarsely chopped *(white/green)*
> 2 stalks celery, chopped *(white/green)*
> 1 medium carrot, peeled and diced fine *(orange)*
> ¼ pound mushrooms, thinly sliced *(white/green)*
> ½ green bell pepper, diced fine *(yellow/green)*
> 1 twenty-eight-ounce can pureed tomatoes *(red)*
> 1 teaspoon dried basil *or* 1½ tablespoons fresh
> 1 teaspoon dried oregano *or* 2 teaspoons fresh
> ½ teaspoon dried rosemary *or* 1 teaspoon fresh
> ⅛ teaspoon ground allspice
> 1½ teaspoons salt
> ½ teaspoon freshly ground pepper
> 1 teaspoon sugar
> 2 tablespoons red wine
> 2 tablespoons water
> 12 ounces soy ground round
> 2 tablespoons grated Parmesan cheese
> 2 tablespoons finely chopped fresh parsley

In a large stockpot, heat the olive oil over medium-high heat. When hot, add garlic, onion, celery, carrot, mushrooms, and green bell pepper. Sauté until vegetables are soft but not browned, about 4 minutes. Turn heat to medium-low and add tomato puree, basil, oregano, rosemary, allspice, salt, pepper, sugar, wine, and water, and stir to blend. Cover and let simmer 30 minutes for flavors to blend. If sauce seems too thick, add water a few tablespoons at a time. Add soy ground round, Parmesan cheese, and parsley, stir, and simmer a few more minutes, until soy ground round is heated through. Serve over whole-wheat pasta.

NUTRITIONAL ANALYSIS PER SERVING: Calories: 247 • Protein: 24 grams • Fat: 5 grams • Carbohydrate: 32 grams • Fiber: 11 grams • α-carotene: 641 μg; • β-carotene: 2,077 μg • lutein + zeaxanthin: 225 μg • lycopene: 33,090 μg

Cabbage and Bell Pepper Slaw *(green; yellow/green)*

This is another beautifully colorful salad. Rather than the mayonnaise-heavy deli-style slaw, this one features green cabbage, carrots, and peppers and has a spicy dressing made with Anasheim chiles. It makes a wonderful side dish for a casual meal of veggie burgers, but I have also served this at Thanksgiving to rave reviews. The next day, you can use the leftovers on a sandwich for a colorful, healthy alternative to lettuce. SERVES 12

1 small head green cabbage *(green)*

2 large carrots, grated *(orange)*

1 yellow bell pepper, cored, seeded, and sliced into julienne strips *(yellow/green)*

1 red bell pepper, cored, seeded, and sliced into julienne strips *(red/purple)*

½ large *or* 1 small purple onion, cut in half, then sliced paper thin *(red/purple)*

¼ cup minced fresh parsley

DRESSING

1 whole canned mild green Anaheim chili

½ cup tarragon or rice wine vinegar

1 tablespoon lime juice

4 tablespoons olive oil

1 tablespoon Dijon-style mustard

2 cloves garlic *(white/green)*

2 teaspoons sugar

1¼ teaspoons salt

½ teaspoon ground cumin

¼ teaspoon tabasco

Freshly ground pepper to taste

2 teaspoons grated lime zest

1 tablespoon caraway seeds (optional)

Core the cabbage, then remove and discard the tough outer leaves. Cut the cabbage head in half and shred into very fine strips. Place in a colander and rinse under very *hot* water, squeezing the cabbage gently until it softens slightly, about 2 minutes. Then rinse with cold water. Working in large handfuls, place the cabbage in a kitchen towel and dry. As you finish with each handful, place the cabbage in a large bowl. When all the cabbage has been rinsed and dried, toss with the carrots, bell peppers, onion, and parsley. Put all the dressing ingredients except the caraway seeds in the blender and blend until smooth. Add to cabbage mixture with the caraway seeds and toss thoroughly. Chill well to allow flavors to blend before serving.

NUTRITIONAL ANALYSIS PER SERVING: Calories: 73 • Protein: 1 gram • Fat: 5 grams • Carbohydrate: 8 grams • Fiber: 2 grams • α-carotene: 409 μg; • β-carotene: 863 μg • β-cryptoxantin 136 μg • lutein + zeaxanthin: 178 μg

Halibut and Vegetable Kabobs

(*yellow/green; red; white/green*)

Fish kabobs make an attractive presentation and are a snap to make. You can thread the skewers and make the basting sauce in advance, and then broil or barbecue. Any firm fish will work for this recipe, as will cubed chicken breast. Vary the vegetables according to your taste, but mushrooms, tomatoes, and peppers are classic. If you plan to barbecue the kabobs and are using wooden skewers, soak the skewers in water briefly before threading so they won't burn. This recipe will make one large or two small skewers per serving. SERVES 4

2 pounds fresh halibut filet
Salt and pepper to taste
½ red bell pepper *(red/purple)*
½ yellow bell pepper *(yellow/green)*
1 yellow onion *(white/green)*
16 cherry tomatoes *(red)*
16 medium white mushrooms *(white/green)*

BASTING SAUCE
8 tablespoons low-sodium soy sauce
4 cloves garlic *(white/green)*
1 slice fresh gingerroot ½-inch thick
2 tablespoons + 2 teaspoons brown sugar
2 tablespoons + 2 teaspoons rice wine vinegar

Cut the halibut fillet into 1-inch cubes, making enough to evenly thread onto 8 skewers. Sprinkle with salt and pepper and set aside. Cut the red and yellow bell peppers into 1-inch squares. Cut the onion into 8 large chunks, and then separate each chunk into two pieces for easier threading. Wash the mushrooms and snap off the stems.

Thread the fish, peppers, onions chunks, mushrooms, and tomatoes onto 4 large or 8 small skewers. If you are not going to cook the kabobs right away, place in the refrigerator, loosely covered with waxed paper.

Whirl all ingredients for the basting sauce in the blender.

Preheat broiler and spray cold broiler pan with pan spray. Place broiler pan under the heat for a few minutes to heat up, then place the skewers carefully on the hot pan. This will sear the fish and vegetables quickly. Spoon some of the basting sauce over the fish, and broil 3 to 4 minutes, or until fish and vegetables begin to brown. Turn skewers, spoon basting sauce over, and cook the other side for another 2 to 3 minutes. Spoon any additional basting sauce over the fish when serving.

NUTRITIONAL ANALYSIS PER SERVING: Calories: 335 • Protein: 52 grams • Fat: 6 grams • Carbohydrate: 19 grams • Fiber: 3 grams • α-carotene: 75 μg; • β-carotene: 490 μg • β-cryptoxantin 204 μg • lutein + zeaxanthin: 80 μg • lycopene: 1,861 μg

Breakfast Burritos (red; yellow/green; white/green)

Burritos are often loaded down with meat, cheese, and sour cream, and wrapped in high-fat flour tortillas. This version features fat-free, whole-grain corn tortillas, wrapped around high-protein egg whites and soy sausage, with avocado and tomato salsa providing a flavor boost. SERVES 2

> ¼ avocado *(yellow/green)*
> 4 corn tortillas
> Nonfat pan spray
> 2 soy sausage patties
> 6 egg whites
> 1 scallion, chopped *(white/green)*
> Prepared tomato salsa *(red)*

Peel avocado, dice, and set aside. Wrap tortillas in foil and place in a 350° oven to heat while you are preparing the eggs and sausage. In a non-stick skillet or a skillet sprayed with nonfat pan spray over medium-low heat, crumble sausage patties and stir just long enough to heat the sausage thoroughly. Remove the sausage to a covered bowl and set aside. Wipe out the skillet with a paper towel, spray with pan spray, and return skillet to the heat. Whisk the egg whites with a fork and pour into the heated pan. Cook, stirring frequently, until eggs are scrambled.

To assemble, place two tortillas on each of two plates. Evenly divide sausage, egg whites, and avocado among the tortillas. Top with chopped scallion and salsa, and roll tortilla around filling.

NUTRITIONAL ANALYSIS PER SERVING: Calories: 310 • Protein: 33 grams • Fat: 5 grams • Carbohydrate: 36 grams • Fiber: 9 grams • α-carotene: 15 μg • β-carotene: 170 μg • β-cryptoxantin 18 μg

Chicken and Brown Rice Bowl

(green; orange; white/green)

This recipe is a healthier, more colorful version of chicken and rice bowls which have become popular quick-food alternatives to the usual burgers and fries. As typically served in food courts, these bowls are heavy on white rice, usually use the more fatty chicken thigh meat, and are skimpy on vegetables. This version features whole grain brown rice, an abundance of vegetables, and chicken breasts. SERVES 4

4 chicken breast halves, boneless and skinless
Salt and pepper to taste
Nonfat pan spray
2 cups broccoli florets, in bite-size pieces
1 teaspoon olive oil
2 cups sliced bok choy cabbage *(green)*
2 carrots, sliced into matchsticks *(orange)*
½ yellow onion, sliced *(white/green)*
2 cloves garlic, minced *(white/green)*
1 scallion, chopped *(white/green)*
2 teaspoons minced fresh gingerroot
2 cups freshly cooked brown rice
Bottled teriyaki sauce

Season chicken breasts on both sides with salt and pepper. Spray a large skillet for which you have a cover with pan spray. Place pan over medium-high heat, and heat for 1 minute. Place chicken breasts in pan and cook for 5 to 7 minutes, or until meat begins to brown. Turn chicken breasts over, cover the skillet, and turn the heat down to medium-low. Allow the chicken to cook in its own juices for another 12 to 15 minutes, or until cooked through. Turn off the heat, remove chicken breasts from the pan, slice, place back in the pan, and cover to keep warm.

While the chicken is cooking, bring 6 cups of water to a boil in a medium-size covered saucepan. When the water boils, drop in the broccoli florets and let cook for 1 minute—just long enough to turn bright green and become slightly tender. Drain broccoli but do not rinse.

Heat a large skillet over high heat and add the olive oil. Add broccoli, cabbage, carrots, onion, garlic, and scallion and ginger, and stir-fry for 3 to 4 minutes, until vegetables are crisp-tender. Season with salt and pepper to taste.

Divide the cooked brown rice into four bowls. Top rice with vegetables and sliced chicken breast, and then with teriyaki sauce to taste.

NUTRITIONAL ANALYSIS PER SERVING: Calories: 332 • Protein: 34 grams • Fat: 5 grams • Carbohydrate: 12 grams • Fiber: 1 gram • α-carotene: 1,235 μg; • β-carotene: 2,414 μg • lutein + zeaxanthin: 1,174 μg

Spicy Fish Stew *(red; yellow/green; white/green)*

This stew is seasoned like a gumbo with bell peppers, garlic, cumin, cayenne pepper, and bay leaves. This recipe is very flexible, and you can experiment with different vegetables, and with a variety of seafood. Frozen shrimp and scallops are widely available and make this dish quick and easy, but you can use any kind of fish. Some seafood markets sell mixed fish pieces for chowders, which are perfect for this and much less expensive than whole filets.
SERVES 4

> 1 tablespoon olive oil
> 1 cup diced yellow onion *(white/green)*
> ½ cup coarsely chopped red bell pepper *(red/purple)*
> ½ cup coarsely chopped green bell pepper *(yellow/green)*
> ¾ cup sliced mushrooms *(white/green)*
> 2 cloves garlic, finely minced *(white/green)*
> 1 cup low-sodium chicken stock
> 2 fourteen-and-a-half-ounce cans diced tomatoes *(red)*
> ½ teaspoon ground cumin
> ¼ teaspoon cayenne pepper
> ¼ teaspoon salt
> ¼ teaspoon freshly ground black pepper
> 1 bay leaf
> 8 ounces fresh or frozen cooked shrimp, peeled and deveined
> 6 ounces fresh or frozen scallops
> 1 tablespoon chopped fresh parsley

In a large soup pot, heat olive oil over medium heat. Add onion, bell peppers, mushrooms, and garlic, and stir and cook for 8 to 10 minutes, stirring frequently. Add chicken stock, tomatoes, cumin, cayenne, salt, pepper, and bay leaf. Simmer, uncovered, for 30 minutes, stirring occasionally. Add the shrimp and scallops to the sauce, cover the pot and simmer another 10 to 15 minutes, depending upon the size of the scallops, until the scallops are cooked and the dish is heated through. Finally, adjust seasonings, remove bay leaf, and stir in parsley before serving.

NUTRITIONAL ANALYSIS PER SERVING: Calories: 215 • Protein: 23 grams • Fat: 5 grams • Carbohydrate: 21 grams • Fiber: 1 gram • α-carotene: 10 μg; • β-carotene: 703 μg • β-cryptoxanthin 276 μg • lutein + zeaxanthin: 82 μg • lycopene: 19,950 μg

Egg White Omelet with Spinach, Onion, Mushrooms, Tomatoes, and Mixed Herbs

(white/green; yellow/green; red)

Omelets are easiest when made individually, so this recipe is for one serving. If you have never prepared omelets with just egg whites, you may be surprised by how much flavor there is. Use a medium-size, nonstick omelet pan with sloped sides for best results. SERVES 1

> Nonstick pan spray
> 1 cup fresh spinach leaves, rinsed and patted dry *(yellow/green)*
> 2 teaspoons minced onion *(white/green)*
> 2 fresh mushrooms, diced *(white/green)*
> 2 tablespoons diced fresh red tomato *(red)*
> 1 teaspoon olive oil
> 4 egg whites, beaten with a fork
> 1 teaspoon fresh chopped herbs *or* ¼ teaspoon dried herbs of
>   choice

Spray the omelet pan with nonstick pan spray. Heat the pan over medium-high heat. Add the spinach leaves, onion, mushrooms, and tomato, and sauté until vegetables soften, about 2 minutes. Remove the vegetables from the pan to a small plate and set aside. Wipe out the omelet pan with paper towel, return to the heat, and add the olive oil, swirling to coat the pan with the oil. Pour in the egg whites, and lift the edges of the omelet as they set, allowing the uncooked egg to run underneath. When omelet is just set, flip it over briefly to cook the other side. Top with the sautéed vegetables and herbs and fold in half to serve.

NUTRITIONAL ANALYSIS PER SERVING: Calories: 135 • Protein: 17 grams • Fat: 5 grams • Carbohydrate: 7 grams • Fiber: 2 grams • α-carotene: 26 µg; • β-carotene: 3,224 µg • lutein + zeaxanthin: 6,715 µg • lycopene: 696 µg

Pita Pocket Tuna Sandwich

(orange; yellow/green; red) (see recipe page 00)

The health-giving benefits of tuna are often undone when it is made into a fatty tuna salad full of mayonnaise. In this version, water-packed albacore tuna is mixed with a tofu dressing, vegetables, and relish to make it lighter and more flavorful and colorful. The whole-wheat pita bread makes a high-fiber container for the tuna salad. SERVES 4

TOFU DRESSING

¾ cup firm tofu
2 tablespoons fresh lemon juice *(orange/yellow)*
¼ teaspoon dry mustard
½ teaspoon salt
⅛ teaspoon white pepper
1¼ teaspoons sugar

4 whole-grain pita pocket breads
1 twelve-ounce can albacore tuna packed in water
2 stalks celery, diced small *(white/green)*
¼ cup finely chopped onion *(white/green)*
2 medium carrots, peeled and grated *(orange)*
1 tomato, diced small *(red)*
2 tablespoons prepared sweet pickle relish
2 cups mixed field greens, rinsed and dried on paper towels,
    then coarsely chopped; or alfalfa or broccoli sprouts *(yellow/green)*

For tofu dressing: Place all ingredients in the blender and blend until smooth (you may need to scrape the sides of the blender with a rubber scraper a few times).

Slice pita breads in half. Drain water from canned tuna, place tuna in a medium bowl and flake with a fork. Add tofu dressing, celery, onion, carrots, tomato, and relish and mix to blend. Then add the coarsely chopped lettuce or sprouts and toss gently. Stuff tuna mixture into pita pockets and serve.

NUTRITIONAL ANALYSIS PER SERVING: Calories: 360 • Protein: 37 grams • Fat: 5 grams • Carbohydrate: 47 grams • Fiber: 7 grams • α-carotene: 643 μg; • β-carotene: 1,507 μg • lutein + zeaxanthin: 834 μg

Sweet-and-Sour Stuffed Cabbage

(green; red; white/green)

Here is another example where soy ground round does a terrific job in taking on the flavors of the dish in which it is cooked. While there are a lot of ingredients in this dish, it goes together fairly quickly and is worth the effort because it reheats well. SERVES 8

1 small head green cabbage *(green)*
12 ounces soy ground round
1 cup cooked brown rice
⅓ cup chopped onions *(white/green)*
½ teaspoon salt
1 teaspoon caraway seeds (optional)
½ teaspoon dried thyme
Freshly ground pepper to taste
2 teaspoons olive oil
1 twenty-eight-ounce can tomato puree *(red)*
½ cup golden raisins
¼ cup brown sugar
1 tablespoon fresh lemon juice *(orange/yellow)*
1 teaspoon rice vinegar
¾ teaspoon salt
1 teaspoon ground ginger

Preheat oven to 350°.

Core the cabbage, and carefully remove 8 large outer leaves, rinse and set aside. Shred the remaining cabbage into fine strips. You should have 6 to 7 cups. Rinse the shredded cabbage and set aside to drain. Bring a large saucepan of water to boil, and cook the 8 large cabbage leaves for five minutes. Cool under running cold water, then drain and set aside. Combine soy ground round, cooked rice, scallions, salt, caraway seeds, thyme, and pepper in a large bowl, and toss until thoroughly blended.

In a large stock pot, heat olive oil over medium-high heat. Add shredded cabbage and cook, stirring occasionally, until cabbage is soft, about 10 minutes. Add tomato puree, raisins, brown sugar, lemon juice, vinegar, salt, and ginger and stir. Lower heat to medium-low, cover, and let simmer 15 minutes for flavors to blend.

While sauce is simmering, fill the cabbage leaves by placing about ½ cup of the filling into the center of each cabbage leaf. Fold up the bottom of the leaf to cover the filling, then fold in the sides and roll up to cover the top.

Place half the cabbage/tomato mixture in casserole dish large enough to hold the cabbage rolls in one layer. Place the cabbage rolls on top, and then cover with the remaining cabbage/tomato mixture. Cover the casserole with foil, transfer to the preheated oven, and bake for 1 hour.

NUTRITIONAL ANALYSIS PER SERVING: Calories: 186 • Protein: 11 grams • Fat: 2 grams • Carbohydrate: 34 grams • Fiber: 7 grams • β-carotene: 467 μg • lutein + zeaxanthin: 279 μg • lycopene: 16,545 μg

Marinated Cucumber Salad (*white/green*)

Marinated cucumbers can be made in a variety of ways, and are always refreshing. This version has an Asian flair, with rice wine vinegar, soy sauce, ginger, and a touch of sesame. The cucumbers will give up liquid and soften as they marinate, so prepare this dish at least 30 minutes in advance. SERVES 4

> 2 large cucumbers *(white/green)*
> ¼ cup seasoned rice vinegar
> 1 tablespoon low-sodium soy sauce
> 1 teaspoon sugar
> ⅛ teaspoon hot red pepper flakes or to taste
> ¼ teaspoon salt
> One ¼-inch-thick slice fresh gingerroot, peeled and minced
> ⅛ teaspoon sesame oil
> 1 teaspoon fresh dill *or* ½ teaspoon dried
> 1 tablespoon chopped parsley

Cut off the ends of the cucumbers. Peel cucumbers, slice very thin, and put in a serving bowl. Mix remaining ingredients in a small bowl. Taste dressing and adjust seasonings to taste. Pour over cucumbers, toss gently, and refrigerate for 30 minutes.

NUTRITIONAL ANALYSIS PER SERVING: Calories: 10 • Protein: 0 grams • Fat: 0 grams • Carbohydrate: 2 grams • Fiber: 1 gram • α-carotene: 4 μg • β-carotene: 8 μg

Chef's Salad with Balsamic Vinaigrette

(*yellow/green; red*)

Typical chef's salads are high in fat and low in nutrition—iceberg lettuce, cheese, an egg yolk, and Thousand Island dressing are the primary components. This version features egg whites and vegetarian turkey for protein, romaine lettuce, spinach, scallions, and tomatoes to help meet your Color Code, and is dressed with a heart-healthy olive oil vinaigrette. SERVES 2

DRESSING
2 teaspoons olive oil
2 teaspoons balsamic vinegar
1 clove garlic, minced *(white/green)*
½ teaspoon Dijon-style mustard
¼ teaspoon salt
Freshly ground pepper to taste

2 cups bite-size pieces romaine lettuce *(yellow/green)*
2 cups fresh spinach leaves *(yellow/green)*
1 scallion, chopped *(white/green)*
2 tomatoes, sliced *(red)*
12 egg whites, hard-boiled and diced
12 slices vegetarian turkey, sliced
2 tablespoons finely minced fresh parsley

About ½ hour before serving, wash lettuce and spinach leaves thoroughly and dry. Place in refrigerator to chill. Mix dressing ingredients in a bowl or shake in a jar, and set aside. When ready to serve, toss lettuce, spinach, scallion, and tomatoes with dressing and arrange on two plates. Arrange half the egg whites and half the turkey slices on top of each plate of greens. Sprinkle with minced parsley and serve.

NUTRITIONAL ANALYSIS PER SERVING: Calories: 305 • Protein: 46 grams • Fat: 4 grams • Carbohydrate: 9 grams • Fiber: 6 grams • α-carotene: 139 μg; • β-carotene: 3,997 μg • lutein + zeaxanthin: 3,163 μg; • lycopene: 3,721 μg

Shopping List for a Week of Color

There's hardly any time to eat in the fast lane that the modern American lifestyle has become. Many of us are eating on the run and don't have the luxury of sitting down to an organized meal. By stocking your cupboard at home, you will have something to eat that is ready in advance to help your health rather than simply add to your waistline.

You don't need to shop every day, but you do want your foods to be as fresh as possible. Most of the foods on these lists will keep for a few days, with the exception of fresh fish. If you prefer fresh fish over frozen, you will need to shop for fresh fish more often, since it should be eaten within twenty-four hours of buying it. The supplies listed below will enable you to prepare the meals outlined in chapter 2.

Shopping List, Days 1 to 4

✔ Meat/Fish/Poultry

Canned, water-packed
   albacore tuna
Chicken breasts
Cod

Halibut
Shrimp, fresh or frozen
Sliced turkey breast, for
   sandwiches

✔ Soy Protein

Firm tofu
Frozen soy
   burger patties
Soft tofu
Soy Canadian
   bacon

Soy ground round
Soy milk
Soy nugget cereal
Soy protein isolate powder

✔ Fruits

Bananas
Berries, mixed (frozen)
Blackberries, fresh
   or frozen

Canned mandarin
   oranges
Cantaloupe
Grapes

Blueberries, fresh or frozen
Mangoes
Nectarines
Orange juice, fresh and
    frozen concentrate
Oranges

Lime
Pears
Pineapple
Pineapple juice
Strawberries, fresh or
    frozen whole

✔ Vegetables

Avocados
Carrots, large
    and baby
Broccoli
Cabbage, green
Cauliflower
Celery
Chives
Cucumber
Green beans,
    fresh or frozen
Green pepper
Lemon
Lime

Mixed salad greens
Mushrooms
Onions, purple
    and yellow
Parsley
Peppers, bell, red,
    green, and yellow
Potatoes
Romaine lettuce
Scallions
Swiss chard
Tomatoes, cherry
Tomatoes, fresh
    and canned

✔ Dairy

Egg whites
Nonfat cottage
    cheese
Nonfat milk

Nonfat mozzarella
    cheese
Parmesan cheese

✔ Grains

Brown rice
Cracked wheat
English muffins,
    whole grain
Rolled oats

Whole-grain bread
Whole-grain
    hamburger buns
Whole-wheat couscous
Whole-wheat pasta

✔ **Taste Enhancers and Seasonings**

Allspice
Balsamic vinegar
Basil, fresh or dried
Black olives
Caraway seeds
Chives
Cinnamon
Cloves
Cumin, ground
Dijon mustard
Dill pickle slices
Dill, fresh or dried
Garlic
Gingerroot
Honey
Ketchup
Mint, fresh or dried

Nutmeg
Olive oil
Oregano
Pine nuts
Red pepper flakes
Red wine
Red wine vinegar
Rice vinegar
Rosemary, fresh
   or dried
Soy sauce,
   low sodium
Tabasco
Tarragon vinegar
Thyme
Walnuts
White pepper, ground

✔ **Miscellaneous**

Canned, mild
   green chilis
Low-sodium
   chicken broth
Olive oil pan
   spray
Prepared
   pizza sauce

Red wine
Rice wine
Sesame oil
Tomato soup
Apricot jam
Cornstarch
Worcestershire sauce

Shopping List, Days 5 to 7

✔ **Meat/Fish/Poultry**

Canned, water-packed
   albacore tuna

Chicken breasts
Shrimp and scallops

✔ Soy Protein

Firm tofu
Soy ground
round
Soy milk

Soy nugget cereal
Soy sausage patties
Soy turkey slices
Vegetarian chili

✔ Fruits

Bananas
Berries, mixed
(fresh or frozen)
Cantaloupe
Kiwi
Lemon
Lime

Papayas
Peaches
Pineapple
Raspberries
Strawberries, frozen
Watermelon

✔ Vegetables

Alfalfa sprouts
Avocados
Broccoli
Cabbage, green
Carrots
Celery
Chinese cabbage
(bok choy)
Corn on the cob
Cucumbers
Garlic
Gingerroot, fresh
Green cabbage

Lemon
Mixed leafy greens
Mushrooms
Onions
Parsley
Peppers, bell,
green and red
Raw spinach
Romaine lettuce
Scallions
Tomato, fresh
and canned pureed
Yellow onion

✔ Dairy

Egg whites
Plain nonfat yogurt

Nonfat milk

✔ Grains

Brown rice
Corn tortillas
Whole-grain bread

Whole-wheat
    pita bread
Whole-grain crackers

✔ Taste Enhancers and Seasonings

Balsamic vinegar
Bay leaves
Basil
Caraway seeds
Cayenne pepper
Cinnamon
Cumin, ground
Dry mustard
Ginger, ground
Hot red pepper
    flakes

Olive oil
Oregano
Rice vinegar
Rosemary
Sesame oil
Sesame seeds
Soy sauce
Teriyaki sauce
Thyme

✔ Miscellaneous

Barbecue sauce
Bread crumbs
Canned low-sodium
    chicken broth
Canned tomatoes—
    plum and stewed
    and sauce
Honey

Mustard
Raisins, golden
Red wine
Relish
Sweet-and-sour sauce
Tomato salsa
Mixed vegetable juice

Now that you have your shopping trip completed, and your kitchen is prepared for the Color Code, you are ready to eat at home in a new and healthy way. Today, that is not enough. With over half of all meals being eaten in fast-food restaurants, from take-out restaurants, and in real restaurants, you will need special skills to navigate your way through what they offer you to eat. The next chapter will give you some key survival skills for the high-fat, high-sugar, low-health jungle out there.

Traveling and Dining with Your Color Code

Whenever you eat in a restaurant, you have to be careful about what you eat and how it is prepared. Yet once you have colorized your diet at home, it is easy to transfer that knowledge to eating on the road and in restaurants.

What does the Color Code look like in a high-priced restaurant? Recently, I ate in a very fancy restaurant in New York while attending a conference. A young physician at our table ordered a big prime rib, French-fried onion rings, an iceberg-lettuce salad drowning in Thousand Island dressing, and for dessert a hot-fudge sundae. He obviously didn't study nutrition in medical school. I ordered a dark-green lettuce salad with balsamic vinegar, baked Dover sole with orange sauce on the side, steamed vegetables, including stewed tomato with steamed asparagus, broccoli, cauliflower, and carrots, and for dessert I ordered mixed fruit, which included kiwi, raspberries, strawberries, and blueberries. I calculated that my meal was over a thousand calories less than his, while going a long way to fulfilling my Color Code for the day. I admit that you won't always be at expensive restaurants, but the idea of getting as much color on your plate remains the same no matter where you eat.

Here are some simple things you can do to stay with your Color Code in most restaurants:

1. If there are chips or bread on the table when you sit down, make a point of moving them as far away from you as possible. A single serving of high-fat tortilla chips fried in oil is over 500 calories, and those wonderful breads and rolls quickly add up to hundreds of calories. If your waiter or waitress tries to serve bread or chips, ask that he or she take your order instead, and take the chips or bread back to the kitchen. At some restaurants they offer crudités, or cut-up vegetables. Ask for these instead of bread if you are really hungry, or have a glass of water or iced tea and make some good conversation until your food arrives.

2. Order a salad with dark greens, not iceberg lettuce. Get as many things added to the salad as possible that provide different colors, including red bell peppers, green bell peppers, carrots, and broccoli. Have wine vinegar or rice vinegar rather than vinaigrette dressings or the usual high-fat dressings such as Thousand Island or bleu cheese. For more taste add small squares or slices of avocado or a touch of olive oil.

3. Order a protein entrée that is low in fat such as chicken breast, the white meat of turkey, white fish, or some other type of seafood. The serving should be the size of the palm of your hand if you're a woman and twice the size of the palm of your hand if you're a man.

4. The size of the protein entrée determines the amount of vegetables you will choose. You should select two different colors of vegetable, or more, so that the size of the vegetable serving is at least twice the size of your protein serving.

5. For dessert, order mixed fruits, such as a bowl of strawberries, raspberries, and kiwi fruit. If these are not available, ask for an orange, an apple, or a pear on a plate. Some restaurants offer baked apples or pears seasoned with cinnamon. Be sure they don't drown them in sugary syrups, then enjoy. Cut any of these fresh or baked fruit desserts up with a fork and a knife and eat them slowly, savoring the flavor as if you were eating a high-fat/high-sweet cake, pastry, or pie.

Avoiding the Big-Plate Special

Don't fall into the "more is better" trap! Restaurants love to serve lots of food. Since most of their costs relate to labor, they think they can get you to come back by serving you lots of food at a low price. If you are eating with someone else, split one large entrée and one salad between you or take home half of your entrée in a "doggie bag." You can save this for a great lunch the next day.

The exception to this rule is the class of high-priced restaurants where presentation is more important than quantity. These restaurants use multicolored sauces to surround small portions of meat, fish, or poultry that are accompanied by beautifully treated but sometimes skimpy amounts of vegetables. However, if you eat at these restaurants, it is usually easy to ask for more steamed vegetables or to order a separate vegetable dish. Continental cooks know the value of multicolored dining.

Restaurant dining should be a pleasurable experience, based on the conversations you have and the people you are meeting. When you walk into a restaurant, visualize sitting down to a fine social experience. It used to be that we ate out only on special occasions such as birthdays or anniversaries. Today, Americans eat out at least 50 percent of the time.

Many times meals are eaten out during the week because there's no time to cook. There might be a special event for your kids, such as a PTA meeting or an athletic event, or you might just have a business meeting that runs late. When you find yourself eating out during the week, don't reward yourself for a hard day's work with a huge meal, or think that you can bury your anxiety by filling your stomach with high-fat foods such as steak and onion rings. You are not a lumberjack, and you shouldn't eat like one. If you need to chomp on something, order a large salad with wine vinegar or lemon and a glass of wine followed by a big plate of steamed vegetables or a vegetable soup. By concentrating on getting your Color Code completed, you will be eating more quantities of food with fewer calories than most foods you can find on a restaurant menu.

Focus on Fat: Restaurant Style

Controlling the amount of fat you eat is another huge hurdle in restaurants because fats are everywhere. You will find fats on the table (butter, margarine, chips), in meal preparation (fried, smothered), and in the ingredients themselves (butter, cheese). Since you aren't preparing the food, learn to ask the right questions about ingredients and preparation so you can get what you want.

  ❖ Ask for fish or chicken to be baked or broiled, not deep-fried.
  ❖ Ask for sauces on the side or ask to have butter sauces left out altogether.
  ❖ Ask to substitute a double serving of steamed vegetables for rice or potatoes.

The International Color Code

Many ethnic cuisines work well with the Color Code because they use lots of vegetables, fruits, whole grains, herbs, and spices. Here is a brief tour of international cuisine with suggestions for menu items that work best.

Chinese and Japanese Restaurants

Chinese foods as they are eaten in China are among the healthiest in the world, but Chinese-American foods are among the highest-fat foods in the world. China has at least four distinct regional cuisines, each one reflecting differences in geography, climate, and historical influences. Szechuan cooks, for example, cook very spicy foods using chili peppers and chili oil. Northern Chinese cuisine emphasizes wheat-based foods, such as noodles and dumplings. In southern China, around the city of Canton (now called Guangzhou), steamed white rice, with boiled or stir-fried vegetables, is made with a minimum of oil. Since many Chinese from the southern provinces immigrated to California in the 1800s, Cantonese food is the basis for Chinese-American foods in which oil and extra-sweet sauces are used. Sweet-and-sour sauce, and the fried dishes drawn from other Chinese cuisines, such as Hunan beef, Szechwan chicken, and shredded pork, were drawn from other areas and repackaged for high-fat American palates. Fortune cookies were developed in Los Angeles by a Japanese-American as a marketing device for the Chinese-American restaurants that dot the American landscape.

Ask your waiter for stir-fried or steamed dishes with a minimum of added oil. Order steamed vegetables and try to get as many of the Asian-specific Color Code items as possible. Bok choy is a great Chinese cabbage dish with a distinctive taste and some of the same protective healthy substances found in broccoli. Most soups in Chinese restaurants are low in fat. Enjoy a cup of wonton or hot-and-sour soup. Go easy on the white rice—limit yourself to about a half cup—and double up on the steamed vegetables while you eat a palm-size portion of steamed fish or chicken.

The Japanese diet is similar to the Chinese, with polished rice, cooked vegetables, pickled vegetables, and seafood as the main ingredients. Soy protein is commonly found in tofu or in miso soup. Sushi bars have become particularly popular and, like American snackables, you can't eat just one. Limit yourself to a set number of pieces. Depending on the amount of rice and fish, women should eat no more than four to six pieces and men no more than six to eight pieces. Have a cucumber salad to start, and a cup of miso soup. Drink at least two cups of green tea. Green tea has compounds called "catechins" that can protect your DNA powerfully.

Apples, plums, red bell peppers, and eggplant are eaten from the *red/purple* group; carrots, winter squash, and sweet potatoes *(orange)* are also used, as is citrus from the *orange/yellow* group. *Yellow/green* and *green* vegetables are widely used, including cucumber, green beans, snow peas, green bell peppers, spinach, broccoli, and cabbage. Foods are seasoned with garlic and onions from the *white/green* group, which also includes mushrooms and asparagus. Asian dishes do not tradition-ally contain foods from the *red* group, although some Chinese-American dishes do contain tomatoes.

East Indian

Cows are sacred to the Hindu people, and vegetarianism is much more common in India than anywhere else in the world. So the East Indian diet is similar to Asian diets and relies on rice and vegetables as key elements. Unfortunately, like Chinese-American food, Indian-American interpreta-tions often have increased fat, added to satisfy American palates. The taste most often associated with Indian food is curry, but there are many others often used in unusual combinations. While many American ver-sions of Indian curry often have added chicken, including dark meat, you can find vegetarian versions and you can ask for light oil or no oil.

Clarified butter (ghee) is the preferred cooking fat, although coconut oil is also used, and foods can be deceptively fatty. For this reason the best choices are tandoori chicken and fish, tomato-based dishes, dahl (lentils), relishes, and kabobs.

Red tomatoes are used in Indian food, as well as *red/purple* eggplant, *orange* sweet potato and mango, *orange/yellow* lemon, *yellow/green* okra and cucumber, *green* cauliflower, and *white/green* garlic and onion. Look for these on the menu or ask your waiter where they are found in different dishes.

Mexican and Central and South American

Most Mexican restaurants make their profits on margaritas, which have over 350 calories per serving, compared to "Lite" beer at about 100 and a glass of wine at 90. They also love to serve oil-soaked tostada chips to snack on before the meal. These have about 550 calories per basket. So you can have 1,500 to 2,000 calories before your waiter even shows up to take your food order.

Mexican food is far more varied than just burritos and tacos. What you think of as Mexican food is probably Tex-Mex. Avoid ordering high-fat quesadillas, taquitos, or Mexican pizza. Chicken or shrimp fajitas with corn tortillas instead of flour tortillas are your best choice. A tostada with grilled chicken is another safe choice if you ask your waiter to eliminate the sour cream, shredded cheese, and refried beans. Substitute salsa for the high-fat American salad dressings that have found their way into these restaurants.

The foods originally developed by the native Indian cultures in Mexico and South America include corn, tomatoes, chili peppers, avocados, squashes, and beans. The red meat, sour cream, added lard in refried beans, and cheese are either Spanish or American additions to a very healthy plant-based diet developed more than three thousand years ago. Cattle were imported to the South American plains from Europe and an Argentinian barbequed beef-based diet has nothing in common with the native diets of South America. Use the Color Code to redesign your plate and reverse history so that you replace these transplanted foods with foods that help you colorize your diet for the day. These foods include *red* tomatoes and salsa; *red/purple* Peruvian potatoes, strawberries, and red wine; *orange* cantaloupe, mango, and pumpkin; *orange/yellow* citrus, including oranges, tangerines, lemons, and limes; *yellow/green* corn, zucchini, and avocados; and *white/green* garlic and onions.

The best choices in Mexican restaurants are soft tacos, fajitas, or tostadas with fish or poultry, whole black beans, and salsas. Some of the more upscale Mexican restaurants offer grilled fish or poultry with salsas made from fresh vegetables or fruits.

Greek, Middle Eastern, Italian, and Spanish

More fresh fruits and vegetables are available in these warm coastal areas than anywhere else in Europe. Fish and other seafood, tomatoes, peppers, apples, pears, cherries, nuts, apricots, citrus fruits, and fresh and dried herbs give this cuisine a rainbow of colors and flavors. Garlic, hot peppers, wild local greens, fresh figs, and melons add spice and taste to meals.

Unfortunately, many of these healthy cuisines are changed when they come to America. Here are some dining tips to keep you using your Color Code:

1. Italian restaurants in the United States are synonymous with pasta and pizza. Both of these dishes have been changed to refined carbohydrates and fat with little to fit with the Color Code other than pasta sauce with added vegetable oil. Order a fish, seafood, or chicken dish with a side order of pasta. Ask the waiter to be sure that there is no oil added to the pasta and order marinara sauces rather than meat sauces on the side. Then you can add the amount you need for taste and you will have a chance to see how fatty the sauce looks.

2. Greek food is also extremely healthy in Greece but not in America. The gyro sandwiches made with lamb and sour cream and grilled onions in oil provide up to 1,000 calories per sandwich. Instead, go for tabouli salad with grilled chicken, fish, or shrimp, and salad with tomato, onions, and cucumber.

3. Middle Eastern cuisine is a general term for Israeli, Persian, and Arabic foods that are not too different from Greek foods. Fried garbanzo bean balls, called "falafel," served in pita bread with lettuce and a sesame oil dressing is the hot dog and French fries of Israel rolled into one. The garbanzo bean balls are

deep-fried in vegetable oil and carry lots of extra calories. Many desserts frequently served in all of these cultures use phyllo dough, which is layered with fat and also carries lots of extra calories.

I have been at Saudi Arabian lunch buffets with huge amounts of high-fat foods. A lot of olive oil and other added fats are used, together with some very interesting fruit dishes including some with figs and almonds. Persian cuisine tends to use a lot of lamb and fish, but also rice with added oil. Use your Color Code to get as many different colors of fruits and vegetables. Taste the many exotic goodies without eating too much of any single dish.

4. Spanish cuisine is famous for paella, which includes pork sausages, shrimp, and fish over rice. Oil is often added to the rice. Once again, try to steer clear of the added fat and calories and order salad, vegetables, and grilled chicken or shrimp.

Order What You Want

Waiters in some restaurants dominate the customers as they recite the mouthwatering specials on the menu. Don't be intimidated. It's not rude to ask how a food is prepared! After all, you are the customer. While you can't reasonably ask for something that isn't even remotely like any item on the menu, you *can* ask for modified dishes—by omitting certain ingredients, or by having dressings and sauces omitted or served on the side.

Become familiar with cooking terms: lower-fat items are roasted, poached, steamed, grilled, broiled, or stir-fried, but "crispy," creamy, breaded, scalloped, or au gratin foods are high in fat. Vinaigrette salad dressings have both oil and vinegar—have them served on the side, not tossed, so you can control the amount you eat.

Read the entire menu, too. Vegetables may not be abundant when served with an entrée, but check the salads, side dishes, and appetizer sections on the menu to supplement your meal and to help meet your fruit and vegetable goals. Ask the server to omit the starchy side dishes and instead double the vegetables. Ask for a chicken Caesar salad without the dressing already tossed in, and have an extra side order of vegetables. You are in charge. The restaurant business is tough, and they need you more than you need them.

Traveling with Your Color Code

It is possible (but not always easy) to stay with the Color Code when traveling. On airplanes, avoid alcohol and snack chips or nuts. Instead, ask for mixed spicy tomato juice, cranberry juice, or water. I usually pack a protein meal bar in my carry-on bag so that when the blue meat arrives, I won't be without an alternative. Even when airline food is decent, I remove all the high-fat items from the plate and put them inside the plastic container that comes with the plastic fork and knife.

When you arrive at your destination, you may find that most stores are closed. Again, a piece of fruit and the protein bar you have packed come in handy. In the morning, most hotels offer a breakfast buffet with fruits. Go for strawberries, honeydew melon, watermelon, and cantaloupe. If you are in a hotel or a motel for several days with no breakfast buffet, keep some fruits and vegetables in a refrigerator in your room. Baby carrots, broccoli, cherry tomatoes, and some berries will tide you over for several days. Buy a few cans of mixed tomato-based vegetable juices in regular or spicy flavors. You can also keep some low-fat meats or soy meat substitutes in the refrigerator.

When you are away on business, you may be taken to some famous restaurants you would never visit at home. Make it a habit to order the specialty of the house with the intention of tasting it and sharing it around your table. Make sure your entrée, salad, and vegetables conform to your Color Code. While some deviations from the plan work, a business trip filled with prime rib, creamed spinach, and mashed potatoes, accompanied by salted peanuts and scotch, will just not fill the bill. While you may have good intentions of making up for your eating when you get home, the next business trip may be just around the corner.

Eating at Family Gatherings
and on Holidays

The holidays can be a great opportunity to introduce your family to more diverse eating and break up some old habits. Here are some suggestions for major holidays:

- ❖ Thanksgiving, Easter, and Christmas. Introduce your family to some new vegetable dishes. Have the white meat of turkey or try a "tofurkey" (imitation turkey breast made of soy protein). Cover these with cranberry sauce containing fresh cranberries. Steam acorn and winter squash, and have some pureed butternut squash. Make salads with multicolored vegetables and use dark-green leafy lettuce rather than iceberg lettuce for the base.

❖ Holiday office parties. Get through these obligatory parties by having a glass of sparkling water on ice, with a lime in it. Then find a talkative person at the periphery of the party and keep your distance from that table with balls of cheese and nuts to tempt you off your Color Code. If you drink, try having a good-tasting red wine rather than hard liquor, and always have some protein such as shrimp, fish, or chicken with alcohol to protect your stomach and balance your nutrition between protein and carbohydrates. Alcohol can inhibit your body's ability to keep your blood sugar up between meals and I have seen people faint by having two drinks on an empty stomach. If you are involved in planning the party, make sure to have cut-up green and red bell peppers (holiday colors, after all) and other colorful vegetables and fruits available at the party.

❖ July Fourth, Memorial Day, President's Day, and Labor Day. The traditional hot dog covered with mustard and relish can be replaced by a soy hot dog. You'll be surprised by how closely they resemble beef hot dogs, and you don't have to worry about what's in them. Grill vegetables on a barbeque, and make shrimp, chicken-breast pieces, or fish on skewers separated by vegetables such as onions and peppers. Skewer two to four vegetables per piece of meat, fish, or other seafood.

❖ Valentine's Day, Mother's Day, and Father's Day. Try avoiding the crush at restaurants and plan a healthy picnic or meal at home using the Color Code you have learned. Center your day around some special activity other than eating. Use the money you save to see a movie or a play or buy a thought-provoking book for your loved one.

Now you have the tools you need to travel and dine out with your Color Code. Remember that vegetables and fruits in the Color Code diet come first, then low-fat protein in about half the amount of your vegetables. Have mixed fruits for dessert. Cakes, cookies, pastries, and chips are off-limits. If you can't eat just one, don't eat any! Do your best to reeducate your taste buds and you will be moving to provide your body with the best pharmacy nature has to offer.

5

Getting Off
the Couch

What does exercise have to do with your DNA? Exercise helps to burn calories and build muscle. Both of these processes involve increased risks of DNA damage, but at the same time both are very healthy. As you take in more oxygen during exercise and burn more calories, your DNA is exposed to more potentially damaging oxygen radicals, but by eating according to the Color Code, you can exercise safely without damaging your muscle tissue excessively. In fact, you will be building muscle more efficiently by helping muscle cells to recover from the stress of exercise.

Building Muscle

When you lift weights you help your health by building muscle cells. The process of building new muscle protein involves nerve signals that are repeatedly sent down to your muscle fibers when you repeat a certain exercise in the proper way. During the stretching part of the muscle action (which would be on the way down for doing a biceps curl), your muscles fatigue. Muscle fibers that normally overlap are pulled apart slightly, sending signals that are the same as those given off by an infection or a tumor, but in this case the signals recruit new baby muscle cells, called "satellite myocytes," and these merge with the damaged muscle fiber to enlarge it. Some damage to DNA within the muscle cells is inevitable, but the damage can be minimized by eating protein after you exercise. It is also important to be eating a diet rich in the antioxidants found in fruits and vegetables to minimize the damage to the DNA in your muscles.

Why bother building muscle if you are going to damage DNA in the process? Exercise is essential to maintain the strength of your bones, your posture, and your ability to achieve and maintain a healthy body weight. Every pound of muscle burns 14 calories per day, so if you gain 10 pounds of muscle you will burn 140 calories more per day. Put another way, you can eat 140 calories more without gaining weight. By building muscle you become more efficient in burning calories, and so you have more leeway in eating to maintain a healthy body weight.

Fitting in Fitness

The easiest ways to increase your calorie-burning activities are simple. Walk up stairs instead of taking an elevator any time you are going up three or fewer flights. Walking after dinner can help digestion and mood as well as burn up calories. Other gentle activities can also be fun things that you love, such as gardening, golf, cleaning your yard, raking leaves, and planting a new tree. Schedule these kinds of activities every weekend to keep your bones and muscles working.

One way to follow your daily activities and make sure you are keeping them up is to use a pedometer. You can purchase one for about ten dollars. These are usually electronic or mechanical devices that count every step you make by having a small part that goes up and down with each step. Whether you are walking up stairs or across a meadow, you will be registering the steps on your pedometer. On an active day, you may register ten thousand steps. Once you have your target number of steps, try to reach it every day.

In addition to these simple things, add thirty to forty-five minutes per day of walking on a treadmill or riding on an exercise bicycle. These steps will also count on your pedometer. Another reason to use the pedometer: Some studies show that after exercising for thirty minutes on a treadmill or a bicycle, you may go easy on yourself and skip walking

your dog or you may just flop down on the couch. As a result, your overall activity for the day may be the same as before you started your formal
exercise program. To keep your heart healthy, it is important to walk in
addition to having a regular workout.

Get Hooked on a Healthy Addiction

These habits are hard to start, but easy to maintain once you get hooked.
I call them the only "healthy" addictions. Start by stretching before you
exercise. Stretching helps to keep your muscles from being damaged during even gentle aerobic exercise. If you don't know how to stretch, get a
book on stretching or ask a fitness instructor to customize some stretches
for you. Then get on a treadmill or a bicycle and warm up for ten minutes, progressively going faster until you get to your target heart rate.
You can calculate your target heart rate by subtracting your age from
220. This is your maximum heart rate. Now divide by 2 to get your starting target heart rate. After a week or two you can increase this by 10 percent. Then after a few more weeks increase the target rate by another
10 percent.

At each point in the process, you should be able to have a conversation while exercising. After twenty minutes at this target heart rate, start
your cooldown and start walking more slowly. If you are on an auto-
matic treadmill or stationary bicycle, it can be programmed to provide
you with a gradual cooldown. These types of equipment are found in
many hotels, and when you are on a business trip, just pack a pair of
lightweight track shoes, a pair of socks, some gym trunks, and a T-shirt.
Then you are all set to relax with exercise while on your business trip.
Anytime you travel for more than a couple of days, a workout like this is
a great idea.

Circuit Training for Building
and Maintaining Muscle

Circuit training is weight training in which you move from one exercise
to another with little rest in between. Going faster and using lighter
weights can improve heart health and endurance, while going more
slowly and using heavier weights can build strength and muscle size,

speeding up metabolism. You can turn any workout into a circuit by going from one exercise to the next with no more than a fifteen- to thirty-second rest period. Repeat the circuit three times for the maximum benefit.

While this sounds like a lot of exercise to be done quickly, you need to concentrate on each movement you are making, especially when you are letting the weight down. This second movement is where your weaker muscles usually come into play and where the damage is done to both the stronger and weaker muscles (called "agonists" and "antagonists" in scientific terms). For example, when you do a biceps curl, the bicep works more on the way up and the tricep more on the way down. The key to building muscle is to feel a burning in your biceps after about ten repetitions and to continue carefully to between twelve and fifteen repetitions. Your triceps will be important in balancing the weight, and if you move too quickly, you can injure your ligaments.

So for each exercise you do, stay focused on the movement and maintain your balance. If you feel out of control, reduce the weight to a level where you can do the exercise correctly. Inflammation of your muscles after an injury will damage your DNA, and that is what you should be trying to avoid. The old adage "no pain, no gain" is simply not true. Pain from injuries to ligaments and joints can permanently sideline you from weight lifting and should be avoided whenever possible.

If you overdo it, rest for a few days until you are ready to resume your routine without pain. While you are healing, use nonsteroidal anti-inflammatory drugs such as ibuprofen, naprosyn, and aspirin to relieve your aches and pains. Use ice packs on damaged joints to reduce inflammation until you are comfortable in a normal range of motion.

There are many different exercise routines you can use effectively, depending on the equipment you have available. I have assumed you are in a gym or have access to one while traveling to be able to do the exercises listed below:

Lat pulldown: This is done with a long bar, usually suspended from a pulley over your head. Space your hands equally apart on the bar and sit down on a bench. Lean back about ten degrees and pull the bar straight down to your breastbone, arching up to the bar as it is about to touch your chest. This exercise builds the shoulder muscles and the upper-back muscles. Do three sets of ten to fifteen repetitions, with only a thirty-second rest period between sets.

Triceps pushdown: The triceps can be built up by pushing down on a gym pulley bar. Grab the bar at a ninety-degree angle to your body and turn your wrist downward as you push down. Don't allow the bar up beyond the ninety-degree angle to your body.

If you don't have a machine available, you can use a dumbbell suspended behind your head. Bend at the elbow until the weight moves down to your back, between your shoulder blades. Now slowly straighten your arm, raising the dumbbell. Do this exercise separately with each arm. Do three sets of ten to fifteen repetitions with only a thirty-second rest period between sets.

Biceps curl: This exercise works best when you concentrate on one arm at a time. Hold a dumbbell in your hand, and without breaking your wrist, slowly move the weight up until your arm is bent as far as it can go. Then lower the weight slowly and deliberately. You will be stretching your muscle fibers on the way down, and it is especially important to go slowly for the last few repetitions of each set. Do three sets of ten to fifteen repetitions with only a thirty-second rest period between sets.

Chest press: This can be done as a bench press with the arms held about shoulder-width apart. With each repetition, slowly lower the bar to your sternum and then slowly raise the weight to get the maximum benefit. If you don't have access to a bench-press machine, a barbell can be used with a flat bench, but you should have a spotter or a special bench fitted with a rack for the barbell. Do three sets of ten to fifteen repetitions with only a thirty-second rest period between sets.

Shoulder press: This is a similar movement to the chest press except that the barbell moves up vertically from the shoulders. Keep your arms shoulder-width apart, and be alert to any discomfort in your shoulders. The exercise is safer with your back supported on an incline bench. If you do this standing, be careful not to use too much weight or to jerk the weight upward. Do three sets of ten to fifteen repetitions with only a thirty-second rest period between sets.

Knee raises: This exercise is performed by lying flat on a bench and extending your legs, then lifting your legs and bending your knees to your chest. This can be done quickly and the number of repetitions increased gradually from twenty to fifty or more. This is a great exercise for the lower abdominal muscles.

Sit-ups and abdominal crunches: Sit-ups are simple to perform and are familiar to most people. Lie on the floor with your knees bent and feet flat on the floor. Put your hands behind your head and slowly raise your head off the floor until you have risen up as much as possible. Lower your head slowly until you are lying flat again. It is important to go down slowly to obtain the maximum muscle-building benefit. Do twenty repetitions initially and increase to fifty or more.

Leg press or squat: This exercise will build the very large quadriceps muscle on the top of your thigh. It will stabilize your knees, and it is the muscle that can best be built up to increase your metabolism. Put your feet in place on the leg-press machine and push away from your body. Start with a comfortable weight and increase each week until you can press your body weight easily. If you don't have access to a leg-press machine, then you will need to do a squat. Hold a barbell across your shoulders and slowly bend at the knees. Tilt slightly forward while holding in your stomach muscles. Do not allow your lower back to bulge backward or you will injure it. If you have any back pain or problems, use the seated leg press so that your lower back is supported during this important exercise. Do three sets of ten to fifteen repetitions with only a thirty-second rest period between sets.

Calf raises: With a barbell held between your shoulders, rise up on your toes as high as you can. There are also machines that have pads that fit on your shoulders while you stand on a platform a few inches off the ground. You can do the same movement, as if you were standing on the floor, more easily with this machine. Do three sets of ten to fifteen repetitions with only a thirty-second rest period between sets.

Planning Your Foods Before
and After Exercise

It is hard to perform exercises when you are still digesting food, and it is hard to exercise if you skipped your last meal. It is important to be careful about what you eat both before and after exercise.

If you eat too much, your intestines will steal the blood flow from your muscles and you will end up getting a cramp. You should not exercise for about thirty minutes after a meal, and you should avoid a heavy protein meal just before exercising.

The best thing to have before exercise is a light meal that combines protein, fruits, vegetables, and some whole-grain carbohydrate. It is not important which fruits or vegetables on the Color Code you have eaten, since the protective substances in your body reflect not just one meal but what you have been eating for days and weeks.

Loading up with carbohydrates is also not necessary if you have been eating normally for the past few days. You are not trying to win a gold medal in the marathon, you just want enough energy for your exercise session.

In summary, no special planning of your meal is required before you exercise, but you must wait at least thirty minutes after eating and you should not overeat before exercising.

On the other hand, after you finish exercising it is very important that you eat a serving of protein the size of the palm of your hand and a small amount of carbohydrate (like a piece of fruit), and that you take in enough water to restore your fluid balance.

Thirst is an excellent monitor of how much fluid you need, and unless you have been sweating profusely during your workout, quenching your thirst with water is just fine. You don't need special sports drinks. To check to see how much water you need, weigh yourself before and then after your workout. For each pound of weight you lose, drink two cups of water. If you don't feel like eating solid protein foods after you exercise, a protein shake or bar is a great way to get nutrition into your system easily. Some companies are marketing muscle-recovery bars designed for this purpose. The protein acts to minimize the pain and burning in your muscles and joints by reducing the breakdown of muscle protein after you exercise.

Eating the seven servings of the Color Code fruits and vegetables every day provides phytonutrients that help protect your muscle cells from damage by oxygen as you exercise.

In addition to eating fruits and vegetables, there are some antioxidant supplements, including vitamin E, that have been shown to reduce damage to muscle fiber following weight lifting. The signals being sent among your muscle cells are the same types of signals involved in infections, tumors, and heart disease. When these signals are traveling among cells, your DNA is subject to damage that can be blocked by the protective substances in fruits and vegetables. In the next chapter you will learn how to use a number of supplements and herbs to help protect your DNA for those times when your diet is just not enough.

6

Supplements: Pills and Foods for Health

For the past fifty years, the accepted medical wisdom (and what I was taught in medical school twenty-five years ago) was that you could get everything you needed for healthful nutrition from the four basic food groups. This has turned out not to be true. In fact, compelling science and bitter experience have taught us that there are some supplements you really do need in order to be healthy, because they are not eaten routinely by most Americans. A serious birth defect, spina bifida, in which the spinal cords of newborn infants are not fused properly, has been shown to be due to deficiencies of folic acid in pregnant women. And a calcium deficiency has been shown to lead to osteoporosis, or a thinning of the bones.

When the typical American diet is examined, it is shocking to find that both folic acid and calcium are not eaten in adequate amounts by most Americans. It's not that you can't find these substances in widely available foods such as dark-green leafy lettuce and dairy products, but rather that Americans simply don't eat enough of them.

Consumers have been way ahead of the medical profession on this one, and have been taking supplements for at least the past twenty years. In fact, vitamin and mineral supplements are the most common nonprescription pills taken in this country, with about 40 percent of all Americans reporting that they take them.

They are not a substitute for a healthy diet, but they will help you achieve better overall nutritional health when combined with the typical "good" diet. In fact, studies show that people who remember to take their vitamins in the morning also remember to eat right and go to the gym. Since you won't eat perfectly every day, especially if you travel, vitamins and minerals will help you consistently get the substances you need for good health.

You have probably read about possible side effects and problems with certain vitamins. At first, it seems out of place. How could natural vitamins be toxic? They are not—when taken in reasonable amounts. The most toxic vitamin is vitamin A, and even for this vitamin, you would have to take five times the recommended daily amount to suffer long-term problems.

Say that you take all you need for the day in pills and then follow a healthy diet. What is the downside? You will only be getting twice, or less, the recommended level of any vitamin or mineral if your diet duplicates what you are getting from your supplements. Your body can easily handle this. For each of the vitamins and minerals recommended, there is a biological rationale and a safety factor that is more than generous. Not only are vitamins safe, but they promote your good health!

As you read this, start with a simple program and build up. If you go overboard and try to take too many pills, there is a chance you will burn out and stop taking the important ones. For that reason, the discussion below follows the order of importance and the strength of the evidence out there for taking particular vitamins, minerals, and herbal dietary supplements.

The Core Group of Vitamins and Minerals

❖ A multivitamin/multimineral pill containing 400 micrograms of folic acid, about 5,000 IUs of vitamin A with half as beta-carotene, 45 to 60 milligrams of vitamin C, about 15 to 30 IUs of vitamin E, 20 milligrams of zinc with 3 milligrams of copper, and a series of B vitamins near the recommended dietary allowance (RDA). This is the basic vitamin pill that has the

RDA levels of all vitamins and minerals. If you take this and eat an equal amount in your diet, there will be no problem.

❖ Vitamin E, 400 IUs. The multimineral/multivitamin pill contains only about 15 to 30 IUs of the RDA recommendation for this vitamin. This is supposed to avoid vitamin E deficiency, but it is not enough for you to gain the antioxidant benefits vitamin E can provide. Between 200 and 800 IUs have been shown to have the greatest benefit on immune function for the elderly and to have antioxidant activity for heart disease prevention.

❖ Vitamin C, 500 milligrams. You can prevent scurvy with only 20 milligrams per day, and the RDA was increased to 60 milligrams per day in part to recognize the benefits of vitamin C as an antioxidant. If you eat enough fruits and vegetables you will get a good amount of vitamin C. The body stores about 1,500 milligrams in total, and you lose about 45 milligrams per day in the urine. By taking more than 250 milligrams per day, you are increasing the body's ability to break down vitamin C and excrete it from the body in the urine as a chemical called "oxalate." Above 2,000 milligrams per day causes kidney stones for some people, but 500 milligrams per day is safe. If you eat fruits and vegetables as recommended, you will get about 200 milligrams of vitamin C. So adding 500 milligrams to this is safe.

❖ Calcium, 1,000 to 1,500 milligrams per day. With aging, the absorption of calcium is decreased. Ancient man ate about 1,600 milligrams per day in plant foods, and we evolved to absorb only a fraction of our dietary calcium. Taking calcium with a meal in the form of calcium carbonate will work well, but with age, your ability to absorb calcium is decreased due to decreased acid secretion by the stomach lining. You may want to use calcium citrate, since this form of calcium does not require stomach acid, and is more efficiently absorbed than calcium carbonate (50 percent versus 30 percent).

So, there are my basic four vitamin supplements to complement the so-called basic four food groups. Someday, all of the vitamins, minerals, and other protective substances you need will, hopefully, be in the foods you eat. Until that day, the dietary supplements listed above are strongly supported by nutrition science. Beyond these few supplements, there are others you may wish to take and I will tell you about those. They are for the more nutrition savvy among you who would like to go beyond the basics.

* Selenium, 50 to 200 micrograms per day in the form of selenomethionine. Many parts of the United States have low-selenium soil, and selenium is important in protecting DNA from oxidant damage since it is essential for the function of an enzyme called "glutathione peroxidase," which converts damaging oxygen-charged molecules to their harmless counterparts. In one study of selenium supplemented at 200 micrograms per day, a reduced rate of prostate and breast cancer was observed in the southeast United States. Since the study was designed to test the effects of selenium on skin cancer, additional studies are now being done to confirm these results.

* Green tea extract capsules, 250 to 500 milligrams containing about 100 to 160 milligrams of EGCG (epigallocatechingallate), one of the polyphenols (very strong antioxidants) thought to be most active. Green tea is made by heating or steaming tea leaves after they are picked. Green tea contains powerful chemicals called "catechins" that are very good antioxidants, but they are lost if the green tea leaves are simply picked off a tea tree and allowed to dry. During the time they are drying, naturally occurring enzymes in the tea leaves turn the leaves brown, as the result of breaking down the catechins (see black tea, below). If the tea leaves are immediately steamed or heated, the process can be prevented, protecting the catechins from being broken down. In some experiments, where the ability to protect DNA from oxidation was studied, green tea was 2,500 times as potent as beta-carotene as an antioxidant.

  Green tea also prevents tumor cells from growing new blood vessels, which is one of the main ways tumors grow and spread in the body. There are many drug companies developing expensive agents for the prevention of blood vessel growth by tumors and these are called "angiogenesis inhibitors." If given to a cancer patient, they would have to be taken for life. Therefore, a natural product that is less expensive makes more sense than an expensive drug.

Black tea is made by allowing the normal oxidation of the tea leaves to occur. These leaves contain some of the same compounds as green tea, and our laboratory is studying the properties of both black tea and green tea. About 80 percent of all tea consumed worldwide is black tea, so it would be important to know whether both will work. The usual recommended dose is four cups of green or black tea daily. However, there are green tea extract capsules that concentrate the polyphenols, with the equivalent of from four to six cups of green tea in a single capsule that has a reduced caffeine content. Any one of these green tea or black tea alternatives could be used as a preventive measure for many chronic diseases, including cancer.

❖ Alpha lipoic acid. This antioxidant has been shown to slow the aging of laboratory mice in research conducted at the University of California at Berkeley. Because it is only found in minute amounts in foods, taking supplemental alpha lipoic acid makes sense. Take 20 to 50 milligrams a day if you are generally healthy; if you are diabetic, you can take from 300 to 600 milligrams a day.

❖ Ubiquinone (coenzyme Q_{10}), 30 milligrams per day. This is really not a vitamin, since it is made by the body. It seems to have a special role in muscle cells, including those within the heart. It concentrates in the particles carrying LDL cholesterol in the blood, and protects the cholesterol from oxidation. This action is helpful in preventing the inflammation in the blood vessel wall that promotes atherosclerosis.

❖ Pycnogenol, 100 milligrams per day. This is an extract of the bark of the French pine tree. The main components are phenolic compounds, including catechins similar to those found in green tea, and condensed flavonoids, including anthocyanidins and proanthocyanidins. These are anti-inflammatory and reduce blood clotting as well as acting as strong antioxidants.

The Color Code of fruits and vegetables you are incorporating into your diet, in combination with the few essential vitamins and minerals, will give you what you need to protect your DNA; additional herbal dietary supplements should be regarded only as the fine-tuning. So first practice getting the diet down. Then add your core supplements. Finally, choose those additional supplements and herbs you would like to take.

Notice, I ask you to choose, given the information you have. It is your right to choose to take these supplements and is guaranteed by law in a bill called the "Dietary Supplement Health Education Act," passed by the U.S. Congress in 1994.

While the supplements listed above are to maintain your health, the herbal supplements listed below can be used to help you with some common ailments that lend themselves to self-care. I would like to give you a brief tour of some of the most popular herbs on the market today. I could write much more, but this is intended as only a brief introduction to the herbal bounty of the plant world. By reading this you will get a general idea of how these herbs could benefit you.

Echinacea

Before antibiotics became popular, echinacea was sold in American drugstores, until the 1950s, for the common cold. It is supposed to enhance immune function. The echinacea family includes the purple coneflower, which grows on the edges of cornfields in the Midwest, but several species of echinacea are now being cultivated for sale as herbal dietary supplements. Echinacea, primarily the roots, was used by Native Americans in the Midwest to soothe toothaches, coughs, and sore throats. Surprisingly, while there are many compounds found in echinacea, the active agents in this plant are not known. The usual dose is 225 milligrams per day of a 6 to 1 echinacea root extract. Since the active ingredients are not known, there is no recommendation for particular standardized contents.

When put into the test tube, various extracts stimulate the function of white blood cells. However, in human studies the results to date have been quite variable. Echinacea bottles warn against using the herb over periods longer than six weeks without a break, but there is no evidence demonstrating any loss of efficacy of echinacea in humans.

Nonetheless, echinacea is safe, while the alternatives, such as strong antibiotics, provided by Western medicine are not only wrongly used but dangerous. Antibiotics are supposed to be used for bacterial infections, where they work well. The common cold is caused by viruses, and antibiotics have no role in this treatment. They do, however, stimulate the development of strains of bacteria resistant to infection. The next time someone gets sick, they might need a new, more expensive antibiotic that can overcome bacterial resistance to the antibiotic that was used needlessly for someone's cold.

Chinese Red Yeast Rice

As an agricultural product listed by the USDA in 1920, this red yeast has been a standard part of the Chinese diet for hundreds of years. It contains substances called "monacolins," one of which is identical to mevinolin (lovastatin), one of the most widely sold cholesterol-lowering drugs in the world over the last twenty years. At pennies per day, this yeast could decrease deaths from heart disease by 30 percent. Not only is red yeast cheaper than cholesterol-lowering drugs, it is also safer. At over 500 times the human dose in rats and rabbits, no toxic effects have been observed. With cholesterol-lowering drugs, both muscle pain and changes in liver function can occur. More science will be needed to show the superiority of this botanical dietary supplement, but I predict it will be a mainstay of heart disease prevention some day. Used as a spice, it can also be added to foods rather than taken as a pill. The usual dose is about 2.4 grams of a rice/yeast powder combination capsule where the weight of the yeast is about 0.4 percent of the weight of the tablet. The amount of the monacolin identical to lovastatin at this dose is about 6 milligrams, compared to the 20 milligrams in the usual starting dose of lovastatin.

Feverfew

Feverfew is a member of the daisy family and is a bushy perennial plant you can find in the gardening section at your local building-supply center. It is thought to be native to the mountains of the Balkans and has been cultivated in Europe for centuries. The herbal use of feverfew dates back at least two thousand years. Laboratory studies show that it inhibits the release of a substance called "histamine," which can affect blood vessels and increase the intensity of migraine headaches. The action of this herb is enhanced if it is present before the test stimulus is given. This observation translates to its use in the prevention of migraine headaches. Parthenolide is the active ingredient, and preparations are standardized to deliver a known amount of this substance. A daily dose of 125 milligrams of the leaf, assuming a 0.2 percent content of parthenolide, is recommended to prevent migraines.

Traditional medicine offers pain relievers that don't address the cause of the problem. The migraine headache usually results from a two-step process. First, stress causes muscle tension in the neck and scalp, which strangles the blood vessels. Second, after a period of strangulation, these blood vessels become flaccid and throb. With each throb, the blood vessel is stretched, resulting in the characteristic throbbing migraine headache. I have seen patients disabled by these headaches, and many others addicted unnecessarily to heavy doses of pain medications. Proper use of this herb could improve the quality of life of many migraine sufferers.

Saw Palmetto

Prostate gland enlargement and reduction of urine flow is a virtual certainty as men age. I once knew a urologist who wrote a paper on the decreasing arc of urine streams in men with each decade of advancing age. Whenever I go to a play or a movie and find long lines of men at the urinals, I try to get behind a younger group of men, knowing that urination is a slower process for men as they age. Saw palmetto is widely used to increase urinary flow and appears to be quite useful for this. I have also had men report that when it works, their sexual performance improves. Whether this is simply due to positive changes in the prostate gland, such as reduced swelling around nerves, or is simply a placebo effect is not established at this time. Western medicine offers drugs that affect the neural messenger chemicals in the prostate to counteract the constriction of the urinary passage that is sometimes observed. These drugs and warm baths usually work. Cold preparations containing pseudoephedrine and other antihistamines should not be taken by men with prostate gland enlargement, as they will only suffer more urination problems due to these drugs, which will constrict the passages in the prostate through which urine flows.

The use of saw palmetto also has a long history. The Mayans first used this evergreen palm native to Florida, South Carolina, the West Indies, and Central America for various indications, including as a poultice to treat wounds and for abdominal pain and dysentery. American

Indians used the berries for food and for the treatment of urinary tract conditions in men. The active ingredients remain unknown, and most manufacturers standardize them to the contents of their fatty acids and sterols. The recommended dose is 160 milligrams twice a day of a 10 to 1 standardized extract of the berries containing 85 to 95 percent fatty acids and sterols.

Ginseng

Ginseng is widely taken for energy and stamina, but it does not have a specific curative action. It is called an "adaptogen," which means that it works with your body to adapt to stressful situations. Chinese ginseng is also called panax ginseng and is different from Korean ginseng. While ginseng is native to the woodlands of northern China, much of the Chinese ginseng we know is grown in the red soil of Wisconsin, where it is a valuable crop.

Ginseng has been used by the Chinese for more than five thousand years. This is documented in the oldest existing written accounts of traditional Chinese medicine. In *Shen Nung's Materia Medica,* written in A.D. 196, it is called "a tonic to the five viscera: quieting the spirits, establishing the soul, allaying fear, expelling evil effluvia, brightening the eyes, opening the heart, benefitting the understanding. . . ." Not a bad prescription for our modern lives. A family of at least thirteen different ginsenosides are believed to be the active ingredients. The usual dose is 100 milligrams twice a day of a 5 to 1 standardized ginseng root extract containing greater than 5 percent ginsenosides.

Siberian ginseng is a different plant but it is also used as an adaptogen. The active constituents are chemical compounds called "eleutherosides." The plant is in the same family as panax ginseng but is native to parts of the former Soviet Union and in certain provinces in China and Korea. It is used in traditional Chinese medicine as a treatment for arthritis, bronchitis, lung ailments, high blood pressure, and high cholesterol, but it is not accorded the same status as panax ginseng. The usual dose is 150 to 300 milligrams twice a day of a standardized 10 to 1 root extract containing 0.8 percent eleutherosides.

Garlic

Garlic is in the lily family, and is considered a food, a spice, and a medicinal herb. Modern garlic probably originated from its wild ancestor in central Asia. It has been cultivated for over five thousand years. As early as 3200 B.C., the Egyptians wrote about garlic, and garlic cloves were found in King Tut's tomb. In India some 2,600 years ago, the medicinal properties of garlic were described. Sulfur compounds, which also give garlic its odor and its nickname of the "stinking rose," account for its medicinal activities.

These sulfur compounds have been shown, in the laboratory, to inhibit the growth of breast and prostate tumor cells. Some studies show that garlic can reduce blood pressure by increasing blood flow in the capillaries, the tiny blood vessels located throughout the body. Effects on cholesterol, which are sometimes claimed, have been difficult to demonstrate in all studies. The usual dose is one clove of garlic per day, or two grams of fresh garlic. Garlic tablets that are coated can prevent stomach acid from breaking down the active ingredients so that they can form farther down in the intestine. The breakdown and absorption of active ingredients from garlic require further study, but the usual recommended dose per day in tablets is 650 milligrams of garlic powder containing a standardized amount of allicin, a compound that is not absorbed into the body but is still used to standardize different garlic preparations.

Ginkgo Biloba

The ginkgo tree is a 150-million-year-old dinosaur of the plant world, and is among the oldest living species on earth. The trees nearly became extinct during the Ice Age, but wild stands of the trees survived in parts of China. Due to deforestation they almost became extinct again, but according to legend were saved by Chinese monks who considered them holy. In this ancient tree species, there are separate male and female trees. The female trees bear a fruit called the "ginkgo nut" (even though it is not a nut). The rotting nuts give off a foul odor, so the female trees are rarely grown in this country. The male tree is grown frequently on streets in urban areas, since the tree is resistant to pests and pollution. The leaves resemble a maidenhair fern and are easy to identify as they have two lobes, thus giving rise to the name "biloba."

Leaf extracts contain ginkgo flavonoid glycosides and terpene lactones, which are thought to be the active agents in ginkgo. There is some evidence that ginkgo can increase blood flow in the brain and improve mental function in the early stages of Alzheimer's disease and other forms of dementia. It can also inhibit platelet-activating factor, giving rise to the recommendation that this herb be avoided by people on blood-thinning agents. Much more work needs to be done to document the exact mechanisms at work here.

Many baby boomers take this herb to enhance their ability to find their car keys. I often find that these people are simply overloaded with tasks and have some minor memory loss. This common form of memory loss usually doesn't respond to ginkgo biloba. The usual dose per day is 120 to 240 milligrams containing 22 to 27 percent ginkgo flavone glycosides and 5 to 7 percent terpene lactones.

Kava Kava

Kava kava has been used safely in Polynesian societies for centuries. Its official Latin name is *Piper methysticum*, meaning "intoxicating pepper," and it was discovered on Captain Cook's second expedition to the South Seas in 1772. In European herbal medicine kava kava has been used for mild anxiety states, nervous tension, muscle tension, and mild insomnia. In Utah, a state where alcohol is restricted, the highway patrol supposedly stops young motorists returning from kava kava parties for driving under the influence. The active ingredients are kavalactones, and these are used to standardize preparations. Kava kava is commonly used as a social beverage in Fiji, and offers relaxation and stress reduction to many westerners who now use this herb on a regular basis for anxiety, tension, and stress.

To the extent that it can be used as a substitute for stronger and more expensive antianxiety and sleep-inducing drugs, it has potential as a self-care option. The usual dose is 70 milligrams of kavalactones in a standardized 11 to 1 root extract one to three times a day for anxiety and muscle tension, and 210 to 500 milligrams of kavalactones one hour before bedtime for sleep.

Valerian

The name "valerian" comes from a Latin root meaning "to be healthy." It is said to have sedative properties, and is mainly used as a sleep aid. It was described by the Greeks and Romans, to whom the plant may have come from northern Europe. Valerian has a penetrating smell that many find unpleasant, similar to sweat socks in a gym. This smell is from a compound called "isovaleric acid" that forms from the breakdown of compounds in the freshly extracted herb, which does not have this smell. However, the smell of the plant is very attractive to small animals such as cats. Legend has it that the pied piper of Hamlen used valerian to lure rats to follow him out of town. In World War I and World War II, valerian was used to treat shell shock. It is still listed in the U.S. and British pharmacopeia as a sedative. The active ingredient is thought to be valerenic acid, and the usual dose is 350 to 500 milligrams of a standardized extract containing 0.8 percent valerenic acid taken forty minutes to an hour before bedtime.

St. John's Wort

St. John's wort has had a reputation since antiquity of being able to offer protection from evil spirits, but in recent times it has been shown to be effective against common garden-variety depression, which is rampant in our society. Since the 1700s herbalists have been using St. John's wort for this purpose, but its medicinal use for wound healing, as a diuretic, and for nerve compression such as sciatica dates back to the time of Galen and Hippocrates in ancient Greece. There are over four hundred species of this plant distributed worldwide. In the United States, this plant is especially abundant in northern California and southern Oregon, from which it derives its common U.S. name, Klamath weed.

There is still controversy on the mechanism of action of this herb. Some texts call it a serotonin reuptake inhibitor similar to Zoloft or Prozac, while other texts call it a monoamine oxidase inhibitor similar to Elavil. Studies being done in our group are attempting to explore the mechanism of action. The active ingredients were once thought to be hypericin, but now there is evidence that another group of compounds, hyperforins, may be the active compounds. The extracts of these little, yellow five-petaled flowers may hold the key to solving some of the most common mental problems suffered by modern man. The usual dose per day is 300 to 900 milligrams of a 5 to 1 extract of the flowering tops and leaves of the plant standardized to contain 0.3 percent hypericin or 3 to 5 percent hyperforin. The minimal treatment time is four to six weeks. This herb is among the most popular sold in Europe.

These herbs are examples of the bounty in nature that awaits our increased understanding of the plant world. In a sense, this is the job the Color Code started. Among plant foods there are many with medicinal benefits. By increasing our intake of a variety of plant foods in our diet and as supplements, not only can we obtain optimal nutrition, but the myriad natural chemicals in herbs may someday help us with the aches and pains of everyday life.

As self-care and alternative medicine spread, they may help modern medicine avoid a looming financial catastrophe in the next ten years. Today we have a mature herbal medicine system in Germany where a book called *The German Commission Monograph E* specifies methods of manufacturing a discrete number of commonly used herbs. Many of the best-selling herbs in the United States are drawn from these. American consumers who have never tried herbs may certainly feel the desire to try to reap some of the benefits they have heard about. But they remain skeptical, in large part due to concerns about safety and also about actually getting the type and amount of herb listed on the labels of these products.

In the next chapter you will learn more about fruits and vegetables, spices and nuts that are eaten less often or in smaller amounts in the Color Code diet but serve to enrich its taste and variety. First, you should concentrate on eating the seven fruits and vegetables we have on the Color Code, but as you go along with this plan, you may want to further diversify your rainbow of colors to include some new and interesting tastes.

7

Discovering the World of Plant Foods

There are 150,000 edible plant species on earth, and we have just listed about 60 or so varieties in our Color Code. While this is a big improvement over the few servings per day the average American eats, there is still a long way to go to get to the over 800 varieties eaten by hunter-gatherers. Plant foods include spices, nuts, and seeds as well as fruits and vegetables. Since it is not practical to eat the volume of fruits and vegetables eaten by hunter-gatherers in the wild, what you eat must be a rich source of healthful chemicals that promote health.

The Color Code begins the job of increasing the variety of nutrients and phytochemicals in your diet, but there are many more phytonutrients out there in spices, nuts, seeds, and unusual fruits. Asian markets have many more varieties of fruits and vegetables than do American produce sections. Traditionally, Asian societies such as Japan and China have eaten persimmons, starfruit, and other fruits we rarely eat. They also eat many different dark-green vegetables, including bok choy and many less well known vegetables, often with only Asian names.

In this chapter you will learn about fruits, vegetables, nuts, seeds, and spices that will enrich the Color Code with more healthy and diverse tastes.

Broadening a Boring Diet

While estimates vary, on average only 20 percent of Americans eat more than five servings of fruits and vegetables a day. While this doesn't sound too good, it is even worse than it sounds. A serving just isn't that big. Here are the official definitions of one serving that broaden what I have already given you as general guidelines:

- 1 medium-size piece of fruit
- 1 cup of raw, leafy vegetables
- three-quarters cup (6 fluid ounces) of 100 percent fruit or vegetable juice
- one-half cup cooked or canned vegetables (including beans or peas) or fruit
- one-quarter cup dried fruit

Market surveys show that most Americans are purchasing the same fruits and vegetables over and over again. In fact, the five top picks for fruits and vegetables are:

- head (iceberg) lettuce
- tomatoes (including sauces)
- potatoes (mainly French fries)
- bananas
- oranges (mainly as juice)

While some of these are healthy, and others provide the taste sensations to bring more fruits and vegetables into your diet, the lack of variety is obvious. Variety and rich diversity are essential to better nutrition. Using the Color Code, you have learned how to begin to broaden your diet to get at least seven different colorful vegetables and fruits into your diet. In this chapter you will learn how to broaden your diet further by selecting fruits and vegetables you may not have eaten before. You will also learn about spices and nuts in the diet.

Try Some New Fruits and Vegetables

Many fruits and vegetables are grown in temperate climates, and you may have to go to specialty stores to get them. California grows 250 varieties of fruits and vegetables, and accounts for 50 percent of the fruits and vegetables exported around the country. Other states and nations listed below also grow these fruits and vegetables, and these are increasingly available year-round because of the opposite seasons above and below the equator, so you should be able to find these in local specialty markets where you live. If there is an Asian market or Hispanic market in your area, explore the produce section and you will find many of the less common fruits and vegetables. Frozen fruits and vegetables and fruits canned without added sugar are other ways you can enjoy some of these no matter where you live.

Avocados

Avocados are best known to most Americans as the key ingredient in guacamole on Super Bowl Sunday, but among fruits they have some unique properties. Their green color is consistent with the fact that they have more lutein than any other fruit, and they also contain glutathione and phytosterol, which inhibits cholesterol absorption. They also contain monounsaturated fat, similar to the olive, and provide a taste boost for other fruits and vegetables. Avocados are also used as a substitute for spreads such as mayonnaise or margarine, and cubed avocados can be used in a salad instead of salad dressings. Avocados were known as "testicle fruit" by ancient peoples in Central and South America and had a reputation as an aphrodisiac. However, there is no evidence that this good-tasting fruit has such extra powers over human behavior.

Avocados are a significant crop in California, Florida, New Zealand, and South America. California, where avocados are extremely popular, produces large quantities annually. The Hass avocado is one of the most popular varieties. Commercial plantings are also in Israel and Spain. As you try different varieties of avocados, you will find different fat and water contents and some very different tastes. The higher the fat content of the particular avocado variety you are trying, the greater will be its taste and texture. The avocado is in the *yellow/green* group already, but is an unusual fruit nonetheless.

Figs Sweeten Ancient Palates

Imagine the world before refined sugar became available in the 1600s, and candy bars in the 1800s. Sweet fruits were highly valued to restore energy. While the fig leaf provided critical coverage for Adam and Eve's private parts in the Garden of Eden, the fruit itself has been highly valued throughout history.

In fact, given its content of carbohydrates and potassium, it probably served as the sports-drink equivalent at the original Olympic games in Greece. As a token of honor, figs were used as a training food by the early Greek athletes, and figs were also presented as laurels to the winners as the first Olympic "medal." Greek physicians claimed that the fig had tremendous restorative powers. I won't go that far, but as a taste enhancer and natural sweetener, figs are a valuable addition to the diet.

Dried figs make satisfying snacks and sweet and flavorful recipe additions. In fact, the fig is reported to have been the favorite fruit of Cleopatra, with the snake that ended her life being brought to her in a basket of figs. The dense, sweet flesh, coupled with its unique crunchy seed, goes well in baked goods, and with meat, poultry, fish, vegetables, and other fruits. Figs can act as a sweetener in a variety of preparations, and are a natural form of added sweetness. In terms of the Color Code, figs are in the *red/purple* group since they often have a reddish-colored flesh.

Guava

The common guava has a fruit with a yellow skin and white, yellow, or pink flesh. These fruits are round to pear-shaped and measure up to three inches in diameter. The pulp contains many small, hard seeds and has a soft musky smell. Guavas are eaten fresh and are also processed into jams, jellies, and preserves. Fresh guavas are rich in phytonutrients and belong in the *orange/yellow* group.

Kiwi Fruits from China to California and New Zealand

The history of the kiwi fruit began in the Chang Kiang Valley of China. Called "yang tao," it was considered a delicacy by the great khans, who relished the fruit's brilliant flavor and emerald-green color. Knowledge of the fruit expanded to other countries in the mid-1800s to 1900s. A collector for the Royal Horticultural Society of Britain sent samples home in 1847, and another sent seeds to England in 1900. Plants were first exported from China to the United States in 1904, and seeds were brought to New Zealand in 1906. Kiwifruit is available worldwide today and is produced in New Zealand, the United States, Italy, Japan, France, Greece, Spain, Australia, and Chile.

Due to California's late fall harvest of kiwifruit, fresh kiwifruit is available to U.S. and Canadian consumers during the winter months, an uncommon time for "homegrown" fresh fruits. With proper storage and handling, California kiwifruit is available for up to eight months, from October through May. The New Zealand season is exactly opposite. The combination of the two harvesting seasons allows consumers to enjoy fresh kiwifruit all year. The kiwifruit is in the *green/yellow* group, and has a sweet taste that has been likened to the tastes of strawberries, banana, and papaya combined.

Kumquats

Kumquats are native to eastern Asia, but they are cultivated throughout the subtropics, including southern California and Florida. They grow on trees that are eight to twelve feet high. The bright, orange-yellow fruit is round or oval, about 2.5 centimeters (1 inch) in diameter, with mildly acid, juicy pulp and a sweet, edible, pulpy skin. Kumquats may be eaten fresh or preserved, or can be made into jams and jellies; in China they are frequently candied. Branches of the kumquat tree are used for Christmas decoration in parts of the United States and elsewhere.

The oval, or Nagami, kumquat is the most common species. It is native to southern China and bears yellow fruits that are about one inch in diameter. The round, or Marumi, kumquat is native to Japan and has orangelike fruits that are about one inch in diameter. The egg-shaped Meiwa kumquat, with sweet pulp and a sweet rind, is a hybrid widely grown in China. In the United States hybrids have been produced with limes, mandarin oranges, and other citrus fruits. Kumquats belong in the *orange/yellow* group.

Lychee Fruit

Lychee fruit comes from the provinces of Kwangtung and Fukien in southern China, and I discovered it in Chinese restaurants as a dessert, the lychee fruit combined with orange or tangerine slices. The fruit looks like a large white pearl and has a wonderful, sweet taste. There is a large brown seed inside the fruit that is not eaten. It is grown in Southeast Asia, Hawaii, Florida, and California. The fruit is covered by a leathery rind that is pink to strawberry-red in color and rough in texture, so this fruit is *red/purple*.

Mango

The mango originated in Southeast Asia, where it has been grown for over four thousand years. Mango groves have spread to many parts of the subtropical and tropical world. Mango trees grow to be sixty feet tall. The mango tree plays a sacred role in India, where it is a symbol of love. Mango leaves are hung outside the front door of Hindu homes and at weddings to confer blessings and to ensure that couples bear plenty of children. Most mangos sold in the United States are imported from Mexico, Haiti, the Caribbean, and South America. There are over one thousand varieties of mango throughout the world. Mangoes contain a digestive enzyme with properties similar to the papain found in papaya, which, when combined with its natural content of fiber, can aid digestion. A three-and-a-half-ounce serving of mango contains nearly 4,000 IUs of beta-carotene, putting it squarely in the *orange* group on the Color Code.

Papaya

Though its origin is rather obscure, the papaya may represent the fusion of two or more species of *Carica* native to Mexico and Central America. Today it is cultivated throughout the tropical world and in the warmest parts of the subtropics. The papaya fruit is slightly sweet, with an agreeable, musky tang, which is more pronounced in some varieties and in some climates than in others. It is a popular breakfast fruit in many countries and is also used in salads, pies, sherbets, juices, and candy. The unripe fruit can be cooked like squash. The unripe fruit contains a milky juice that has a protein-digesting enzyme known as "papain," which greatly resembles the animal enzyme pepsin in its digestive action. This juice is used in the preparation of various remedies for indigestion and in the manufacture of meat tenderizers. The very juicy flesh of the papaya is deep yellow or orange to salmon colored. Along the walls of its large central cavity are attached the numerous round, wrinkled black seeds, which are the size of peas. The papaya's phytonutrients and color put it in our *orange* group.

Passion Fruit

The purple passion fruit is native in areas from southern Brazil, through Paraguay, to northern Argentina. The yellow form may be of unknown origin, or is perhaps native to the Amazon region of Brazil, or may be a hybrid. In Australia the purple passion fruit was flourishing and partially cultivated in coastal areas of Queensland before 1900. In Hawaii seeds of the purple passion fruit, brought from Australia, were first planted in 1880, and the vine came to be popular in home gardens. The nearly round or ovoid fruit is one and a half to three inches wide, has a tough rind that is smooth and waxy, and ranges in hue from dark purple with faint, fine white specks to a light yellow or pumpkin color. Within is a cavity more or less filled with an aromatic mass of double-walled, membranous sacs containing orange-colored, pulpy juice and as many as 250 small, hard, dark brown or black seeds. Its unique flavor is appealing—musky, guava-like, and sweet/tart to tart. The yellow form has generally larger fruit than the purple, but the pulp of the purple is less acid, richer in aroma and flavor, and has a higher proportion of juice (35 to 38 percent). Numerous hybrids have been made between the purple and the yellow passion fruit, often yielding colors and other characteristics intermediate between the two forms. The purple passion fruit goes into our *red/purple* group, while the yellow variety goes into the *yellow/orange* group.

Persimmons

The Oriental persimmon, an important and extensively grown fruit in China and Japan, where it is known as kaki, was introduced into France and other Mediterranean countries in the nineteenth century and grown, to a limited extent, there. Introduced into the United States a little later, it is now grown commercially on a small scale in California and in the Gulf states, mainly in home gardens. Two main types of persimmon are sold in California. There is the flat, crunchy Fuyu and the acorn-shaped Hachiya. However, there are hundreds of varieties, and the persimmon holds the same place in the Japanese culture as the apple does in ours. A comprehensive collection of persimmon trees at UCLA was cut down in 1960 to make way for the UCLA Medical Center where I work. In the 1920s in California, growers offered dozens of rare varieties of persimmons for sale.

The fruit, five to eight centimeters (two to three inches) or more in diameter and yellow to red in color, somewhat resembles a tomato in appearance. The Hachiya variety, the leading variety exported to East Coast markets, tends to be bitter until soft-ripe. The Fuyu variety is sweeter and snackable, and its growth has been booming since the Asian immigration to California in the 1970s and 1980s. The native American persimmon grows from the Gulf states north to central Pennsylvania and central Illinois. The fruit is up to two inches in diameter, usually rather flattened, and dark red to maroon in color. Most fruits contain several rather large, flattened seeds. The American persimmon's fruit is generally considered more flavorful in its softened state than the Oriental species, and considerable quantities are gathered from the wild. A number of superior kinds have been named and propagated and are grown commercially.

Persimmons are eaten fresh as a dessert fruit, often with sugar or liqueur, or are stewed or cooked as jam. Persimmons are in the *orange* group due to their carotene content, and are also a good source of vitamin C.

Pomegranates: A Fruit of the Old Testament

The pomegranate is native from Iran to the Himalayas in northern India and has been cultivated and naturalized over the whole Mediterranean region since ancient times. Because of its thick skin, it was not interbred extensively and is thought to be relatively unchanged since biblical times. It is widely cultivated throughout India and the drier parts of Southeast Asia, Malaya, the East Indies, and tropical Africa. The tree was introduced into California by Spanish settlers in 1769. In this country, mainly in the drier parts of California and Arizona, it is grown for its fruit.

The fruit can be eaten out of hand by deeply scoring it vertically several times and then breaking it apart. The clusters of juice sacs are then lifted out and eaten. The sacs also make an attractive garnish when sprinkled on various dishes.

Pomegranates are most often consumed as juice and can be juiced in several ways. The sacs can be removed and put through a basket press, or the juice can be extracted by reaming the halved fruits on an ordinary orange juice squeezer. Another approach starts with warming the fruit slightly and rolling it between the hands to soften the interior. A hole is then cut in the stem end, which is placed on a glass to let the juice run out, with the fruit being squeezed from time to time to get all the juice. The juice can be used in a variety of ways: as a fresh juice; to make jellies, sorbets, or cold or hot sauces; and to flavor cakes, baked apples, and so on. Pomegranate syrup is sold commercially as grenadine. The juice can also be made into a wine. The pomegranate fits into the *red/purple* group on the Color Code.

Starfruit

Portuguese traders introduced this uniquely shaped fruit to Africa and South America from India. This yellow fruit is shaped like a five-pointed star when cut in a cross section. It is also known as carambola, which is a Portuguese word meaning "food appetizer." In Malaysia starfruit is grown extensively, with over 48,000 tons of starfruit being produced in Malaysia, and over 11,000 tons is exported from elsewhere. This fruit is starting to appear in specialty produce sections in grocery stores in certain parts of the United States. Starfruit belongs in the *yellow/orange* group.

Watercress

Watercress is an herb in the mustard family and is most famous for its inclusion in watercress sandwiches, eaten by matrons at afternoon tea. Watercress originated in the Middle East. Generals in ancient Greece and Persia ordered their soldiers to eat watercress to keep them healthy.

By the seventeenth century watercress soup in particular had gained a very good name in England. Nicholas Culpeper, in his *Compleat Herbal* writes that cress soup was a good remedy for cleansing the blood in the spring and helping headaches. Watercress is used as a garnish and in salads. Watercress should be stored in the refrigerator with its stems in water and the leaves loosely covered with a plastic bag. Most westerners eat watercress raw. In the East it is blanched, the moisture is wrung out, and then it is chopped and tossed with a light sesame oil dressing. The Chinese often stir-fry it with a little salt, sugar, and wine or use it in soups. Watercress contains isothiocyanates, the phytochemicals that predominate the green group, and so fits into the *green* group on the Color Code.

You Ain't Seen Nothin' Yet

There are many more unusual fruits and vegetables, but this chapter serves as only an introduction to the possibilities. I could literally fill a book by simply describing plant foods you have not eaten, but I won't try here. Beyond the varieties discussed above, there are cultivars, special strains formed by the interbreeding of compatible plants. As you can see, the variations are endless and the variety overwhelming. How much variety is enough? As we learn more about the human genome, we will learn how much variety is optimum, but the Color Code is definitely a step in the right direction.

Herbs and Spices You Can Grow or Collect

Just as the watercress can provide important chemicals to the diet, there are many other household herbs, such as tarragon, oregano, chives, dill, mint, thyme, parsley, rosemary, and sage, that provide unique variety to the diet—not only in terms of taste, but by adding uniquely beneficial chemicals to your diet. Herbs can be used instead of salt to enhance the flavor of many foods. Low-fat cooking methods often require more seasoning to keep food flavorful; herbs can satisfy this need without adding calories. You can buy an herb collection that is dried or you can grow and harvest your own fresh herbs.

Growing Your Own Herbs

In general, herbs do best when grown in sunny areas and in good soil. Most herbs can't withstand cold temperatures, and may have to be grown indoors in many parts of the country. Outdoor gardens should be planted in the spring and weeded often. Indoors, you should use containers large enough to allow root growth and proper drainage. Place them in a sunny area, such as a kitchen windowsill, and water them often.

Most herbs (especially chives, mint, and tarragon) can be divided or cut to grow new plants. To harvest herbs, simply snip leaves or stems with scissors around the top and the center of the plant. Rinse cuttings under cool water and pat dry with a paper towel.

Basil

Basil was considered a sacred herb in ancient Italy and France. Women were not allowed to pick it. Only male religious leaders were allowed to gather basil in a special ritual. Basil plants grow to a height of approximately two feet. To encourage bushy growth, pinch off the flower buds as they appear. As a seasoning, basil is best used fresh. It loses most of its flavor when dried, but dried basil is sold as an herb. Use basil in tomato sauces, pesto, and fish dishes. Basil adds flavor to fresh or cooked vegetables.

Chives

Chives have been enjoyed fresh since the time of the ancient Greeks. The gentle onion flavor of chives adds flavor to soups, sauces, and salads. Since they are so similar to onions and garlic, they are already part of the *white/green* group on the Color Code.

Dill

The Romans believed dill built strength when added to foods. Consequently, gladiators were given food covered with dill to fortify them in preparation for their bloody contests. Dill tends to grow quickly and does not last very long. If you try growing this herb, you may have to plant more dill every two to three weeks throughout the spring and summer. Dill is best known for its use in making pickles, but it can be used in sauces and salads as well. It's particularly good on fish and vegetables.

Mint

There are twenty varieties of mint, including several that grow wild. Most Americans are familiar with these as flavors of chewing gum and hard candies such as peppermint, spearmint, and wintergreen. Bergamot, which is the flavor of Earl Grey tea, is also a mint. Peppermint aids digestion by relaxing the sphincter muscle between the swallowing tube (esophagus) and the stomach, releasing trapped gas after a big meal. That's why many restaurants traditionally serve after-dinner mints and why many antacids contain mint. This is a hardy, perennial plant, and unless it is pruned frequently, it can easily take over a whole garden. You may want to keep it in its own container. Use mint as a garnish and a flavoring for drinks, soups, sauces, salads, and desserts, especially fruit sorbets. It's good either fresh or dried.

Oregano

Oregano originated in the eastern Mediterranean. It became popular in this country after World War II, when soldiers who'd been stationed in Italy brought it home to flavor pasta sauces and other Italian foods. Individual stems or leaves and flowers can be picked off and dried for future use. Oregano is a classic seasoning for Italian, Greek, and Mexican dishes. It also can add interest to many different kinds of vegetable salads.

Parsley

Parsley is the common name for a member of the large family of herb plants containing many important foods and flavorings. There are about three thousand species belonging to the family called *Apiaceae*, of which parsley is one genus. The five-parted flowers are rather uniform throughout the family. The fruits, however, which develop from the two-parted ovary, which is below the leaves, are quite varied. Members of the family include carrots, parsnips, celery, dill, fennel, caraway, anise, and coriander. Some species, such as hemlock, are poisonous. Many other species have been used as medicinal herbs. Parsley plants grow slowly, so they should be weeded carefully until established.

Parsley reaches to a height of about twelve to sixteen inches, and grow well indoors and out. There are two varieties of parsley: curly-leafed and flat-leafed. Flat-leafed parsley has the stronger flavor. Use parsley as a garnish and as a flavoring for sauces and soups. Parsley is a rich source of vitamin C, and can be used to cover up the flavor of garlic. Parsley oil is sold in capsules as a treatment for bad breath after meals. As a seasoning it enlivens the flavors of many bland foods. Try sprinkling it on vegetables or adding it as a colorful garnish to any dish.

Rosemary

Rosemary was a favorite plant in the Middle Ages, not only for its supposed medicinal value but as a symbol of the declaration of love. Rosemary is actually an evergreen shrub. It's sensitive to cold temperatures, and when grown indoors, misting the foliage twice a week is recommended. Rosemary has a distinctive taste due to its content of a phytochemical called "carnosic acid." This phytochemical has been shown in laboratory experiments to combine with other phytochemicals, such as lycopene, from tomatoes, to kill cancer cells. Use rosemary on baked chicken breasts, but go easy, as it has a strong flavor. Rosemary is best dried, and keeps well in a sealed jar.

Sage

Tradition holds that sage is supposed to be harvested on the dawn of Midsummer Day when the first ray of sunlight strikes the highest mountain. There is no scientific reason for this, and sage is picked whenever the plant is fully grown to a diameter of about thirty-six inches. A well-maintained plant will last for more than five years. Dried sage is preferred over fresh sage. Sage is good in tomato soups and with poultry.

French Tarragon

Tarragon is native to northern Asia and not France, as its name would imply. It is best to plant it in its own container, since it can take over a garden. Fresh tarragon is better than dried, and can be purchased in some grocery store produce sections. The only edible part is the leaves. Try tarragon on chicken, with mushrooms, and in soups and sauces.

Thyme

This herb gives off a strong fragrance. It was grown in monastery gardens in France, Spain, and Italy during the Middle Ages for use as a cough remedy and digestive aid. A solution of thyme's most active ingredient, thymol, is used in cough drops and vapor rubs for colds. Thyme plants hug the ground and tend to spread. They generally require minimal watering. Thyme, like many herbs, is also available in dried form, and can be used to flavor soups and sauces.

Pepper, Chili Peppers, and Chili Oils

Peppers have been found in prehistoric remains in Peru. They were widely grown in Central and South America well before Columbus arrived and took pepper seeds back to Spain in 1493. The genus *Capsicum* comprises all the varied forms of fleshy-fruited peppers grown as herbaceous annuals—the red, green, and yellow peppers rich in vitamins A and C that are used in seasoning and as a vegetable food. Hot peppers, used as relishes, pickled, or ground into a fine powder for use as spices, derive their pungency from the compound capsaicin, a substance characterized by acrid vapors and a burning taste, that is located in the internal partitions of the fruit. First isolated in 1876, capsaicin stimulates gastric secretions and, if used in excess, causes inflammation. Hot varieties, which are red when mature, include the tabasco, which is commonly ground and mixed with vinegar to produce a hot sauce, and the long "hot" chili and cayenne peppers often called "capsicums." Cayenne pepper, said to have originated in Cayenne, French Guiana, is one of the spices derived from these peppers and is produced in many parts of the world.

The mild bell or sweet pepper plants have larger, variously colored but generally bell-shaped, furrowed, puffy fruits that are used in salads and in cooked dishes. They lack the gene for making capsaicin and so are not hot at all. These varieties are usually harvested when bright green in color—before the appearance of red or yellow pigment—about sixty to eighty days after transplanting. However, the red and yellow varieties are also usually sold at a higher price than the green bell pepper. The red bell pepper is a good source of vitamin C.

The term "pimiento," from the Spanish for "pepper," is applied to certain mild pepper varieties possessing a distinctive flavor but lacking in pungency; these include the European paprikas, which include the paprika of commerce, a powdered red condiment that was known in Hungary by the late sixteenth century. "Pimiento," often pronounced the same as "pimento," should not be confused with the latter, which is allspice.

Pepper plants are tender summer annuals outside their native habitat. They are propagated by planting seed directly in the field or by transplanting seedlings started in greenhouses or hotbeds after six to ten weeks. Chili peppers are available as mild, hot, and very hot. There is even a scale for rating the hotness of chili peppers. This hotness is actually a pleasant sensation once you are accustomed to it. Scientists have detected increases in the pleasure hormone, endorphin, right after individuals who like to eat chili peppers have ingested them. They also cause sweating and some increase in metabolic rate. Some studies have shown a slight amount of weight loss in individuals who eat hot peppers. They can be used to increase the taste of low-fat recipes.

Be a Little Bit Nuts

There is no question that nuts can be fattening. Eaten by the handful, they add lots of extra calories to an already high-fat diet. However, in countries where nuts are a significant source of calories, the diets tend to be rich in plant foods and low in calories.

Since moving to Southeast Asia would be disruptive for you, the way to use nuts in an American diet is to substitute them for something else rather than simply adding them to your diet. Eaten in moderation as a taste enhancer, nuts can be part of a healthful diet. Not only are they flavorful, but ounce for ounce, nuts are full of nutrients. Most nuts are seeds of the dried fruit from trees.

A Peanut Is Not a Nut

Peanuts, which are commonly thought of as nuts, are actually legumes. They belong to the same family as peas and beans. Because nuts come from plants, they're naturally cholesterol-free. Although nuts are high in calories for their size, they're also considered to be a "nutrient-dense" food. They contain a lot of nutrients in relation to their calories.

Nuts Have Phytochemicals, Minerals, and Good Fats

Some nuts are good sources of thiamin, niacin, phosphorus, zinc, and folate, and some are excellent sources of selenium, copper, magnesium, manganese, and vitamin E. Nuts are also rich in different plant compounds. Flavonoids, for instance, are found in all nuts. These antioxidants help reduce the formation of substances in the body that may contribute to cancer and cardiovascular disease. Relative to their size, nuts are also among the best plant sources for protein.

Nuts are generally high in fat. In most cases, more than 75 percent of their calories comes from fat. One exception is chestnuts, which have only 8 percent of their calories from fat. Most of the fat in nuts is monoun-saturated and polyunsaturated. Unlike saturated fats (typically found in red meats and dairy products), these fats don't appear to increase blood cholesterol. In small amounts, monounsaturated and polyunsaturated fats may actually lower cholesterol. Walnuts and almonds are rich sources of omega-3 fatty acids, but don't get too much of a good thing. Nuts can have hundreds of calories in a handful, and all oils are 140 calories per tablespoon.

There Will Never Be a Nut Diet Book

Nuts are high in calories due to their high fat content. So if you're trying to maintain your current weight, you can't simply add nuts to your diet without expecting to add weight. Instead, you might try to eat them in place of other foods. One way to do that is to substitute nuts for some meat. For instance, one ounce of nuts can take the place of one ounce of meat. Nuts are considered part of the meat group on the USDA pyramid, where they are thought of as a protein source without regard for their high fat content. On the California cuisine pyramid on p. 226, they are taste enhancers at the top of the pyramid instead of oils and sugar, and in my view they should be used as needed to add taste to other foods. If you're a snacker, count nuts out rather than eating them by the handful. One ounce of dry-roasted cashews—about eighteen cashews—has around 165 calories. Toasting slivered almonds or cashews enhances the nutty taste and can add a lot of flavor to a vegetable dish with few extra calories. No more than one ounce per day is the rule for nuts unless you burn so many calories each day that you don't have to worry at all about calories.

Just a Beginning

This chapter is just a brief introduction to the world of plant foods that include nuts, herbs, and spices. Using this as a starting point, you can begin to explore the diversity of the world of plant foods. There are recipes in chapter 3 that you can try. Remember to start with the basics and add these additional foods to your plan slowly so that you can substitute them for other foods instead of just adding them. Too much of a good thing can be bad for you, and that is especially true of taste enhancers such as nuts, since they carry extra calories with them. With fruits and vegetables you will usually fill up before you bulk up, but use your common sense as you explore the world of plant foods. In the next chapter you will learn the truth about fifteen of the most common nutrition myths, which will help put all that you have learned so far into proper perspective.

Fifteen of the Most Common Myths About Nutrition

At times, when I finish telling my patients what to eat, they challenge me with a piece of information they heard from a friend or even their doctor that disagrees with what I have told them. I always take the time to respond in detail, since this gets me closer to my patient's belief systems and increases their motivation to change. It is great to learn new positive information, but you demonstrate your ability to use that new information when you compare your own knowledge with the myths you may have heard. You can use the examples below in answer to questions from your friends and family as you take on this new nutrition plan.

Why Is There So Much Confusion About Food?

Why is it that there is so much confusion about nutrition? We all eat, and so we feel that we should all know what is right. Is it the media, the self-proclaimed overnight diet experts, or our own wishful thinking that perpetuate myths about foods? If you are eating what tastes good to you, it is tempting to think that it is also good for you. It is tempting to think that if only you changed just one thing, you could keep eating the way you have been. You could justify this line of thinking and think you wouldn't need to change a thing.

This book is about changing your whole diet. I don't want you to just cut out the so-called bad foods, I want you to add health back into your diet. So let's start by setting you straight about all the easy wrong answers you have heard over the years.

Myth #1
All You Need to Do to Lose Weight Is to
Eat Less of Your Favorite Foods

This idea is capsulized in the old joke which says that you can't lose weight by talking about it, you have to shut your mouth! In fact, simply eating less of your favorite foods is a very ineffective way to lose weight unless you are a very tall man or woman burning well over 2,500 calories per day. If you burn this large number of calories, any diet in which you cut your portion sizes will work temporarily. If you burn only 1,500 calories per day and try losing weight with this method, you will be frustrated by a very slow weight loss.

Ultimately, as you give in to just one episode of overeating when your stress builds up, you will reverse the progress you have made in a whole week of being careful. Even for the braggadocious big man who loses twenty pounds using the 50 percent method, where he simply cuts his steak in half, my experience is that ultimately he will gain back his weight when the next crisis comes up. The real challenge for you is to permanently change your eating habits by changing the types of foods you are eating, not just the amounts. Losing weight is not the only goal; losing weight in a healthy way so that you include the fruits and vegetables in the Color Code is the way to protect your DNA and lose weight at the same time.

Myth #2
Cutting Out All the Fat in Your Diet Is All
You Need to Do

For almost ten years nutrition experts pushed the idea of simply cutting out fat as the way to lose weight. In the 1980s there was near unanimity among weight-loss experts based on the fact that countries whose populations ate a low percentage of fat calories had less heart disease, cancer, and diabetes. The surgeon general of the United States, in 1988, said that after cutting out smoking the most important thing Americans could do to improve their health would be to reduce the intake of fat in the diets. The food industry believed the experts and came out with over a thousand fat-free or reduced-fat foods.

Two things happened. First, many of the "fat-free" foods had the same number of calories as their regular full-fat versions, since the manufacturers simply replaced fat with sugars. The expected reduction in calories never happened, so there was no effect on body weight. Second, studies showed that if consumers were "good" at one meal and ate fat-free foods, they would allow themselves to splurge at other meals. Once again, no weight loss occurred.

Fruits and vegetables are not fat-free, but they are filling and have fewer calories per bite than similarly sweet sugary treat foods. By adding fruits and vegetables to your diet, you will be displacing the higher-calorie snack foods, such as cakes, pastries, and chips, that are adding unnecessary calories to your diet.

Myth #3
Cutting Out All the Sugar in Your Diet Is
All You Need to Do

As a reaction to Myth #2, other diets claimed that all you needed to do was to cut out refined sugar and flour foods, which came to be called bad "carbs." This simple approach had the advantage of leaving all the good-tasting rump roasts, burgers, ribs, and cheeses in the diet while eliminating the breads and sweet desserts. If breads, pies, cakes, and pastries are the extra calories in your diet that you eat for pleasure or when you are stressed, then you will lose some weight for a period of time. For those people who just couldn't do the low-fat thing, this diet was a godsend for a period of time. They lost twenty or so pounds, but once again regained weight as they eventually added back the refined "carbs" they had once reviled.

The very best thing about this approach is also its undoing. As you keep all your favorite high-fat meats and cheeses in your diet, you never lose your taste for these foods. So when you add back the carbohydrates, you regain all your lost weight. Instead, by using the Color Code, you will be changing the balance of foods in your diet. Not all carbohydrates are created equal. Fruits and vegetables are good carbohydrates, and they provide you with a virtual pharmacy of healthy substances only found together in fruits and vegetables. By adding color to your diet, you add in substances that protect your DNA, fill you up with fewer calories, and provide healthy fiber.

Myth #4
Eating Too Few Calories Will Cause Your Body to Go into Starvation Mode and You Will Stop Losing Weight

This is simply not true. During a diet, the most your body's metabolism is capable of adapting is about 15 percent of total calories burned. So if you normally burn 1,500 calories per day, your metabolism during a very low calorie diet that provides 800 calories per day would decrease by 225 calories per day to 1,275 calories per day. You would have a daily calorie balance of minus 475 calories per day, which would cause about one pound of weight loss per week. There is no question that the rate of weight loss slows down as you approach your target weight, but this is predictable and has nothing to do with going into a state of starvation. One of the key principles you will learn in this book is that you are an individual, with your own best target weight based on how much muscle you were born with and whether you are male or female. It's not overweight but overfatness that defines obesity. When commercial diet programs give out unrealistic target weights based on some insurance company table, they set you up for failure if you have more muscle than the average person. When you reach your own target weight but are still well above their chart ideal, your weight loss will stop and you will go into starvation mode. However, your body is right, not your mind. You are at your target weight or near it whether you want to admit it or not.

Myth #5
High-Protein Diets Cause Ketosis,
Which Reduces Hunger

Ketone bodies are formed from fat as an energy source during starvation. They are burned by the muscles and replace critical carbohydrates, enabling you to starve for months as long as there is adequate fluid intake. So if you eat a carbohydrate-free diet, your ketone bodies will increase as your body tries to burn the fat you are eating in that steak that is the cornerstone of your "high protein" diet. They will turn your breath a bad "fruity" odor, and if you were to use the urine test strips designed for diabetics, they would turn blue when you excreted ketone bodies in your urine. Seeing the strip turn blue is a gratifying experience for the high-protein dieter, as the metabolic "truth" of their approach is confirmed. I hate to burst your bubble, but ketone bodies don't reduce appetite one bit. When infused into humans they don't counteract normal hunger. In this book you will learn to put colors in the foods you eat, not on a plastic strip used to test your urine ketones.

Myth #6
All You Need to Do Is Exercise to Lose
Weight, Since Diets Don't Work

I am a great proponent of exercise, and it is one of the best ways to maintain a healthy body weight once you have lost weight. If you exercise three times a week and get your heart rate up for about twenty or thirty minutes each time, you will be hooked. The blood levels of the hormone endorphin will rise in anticipation of your exercise session and you will feel deprived if you don't get a chance to exercise. In fact, it is the only healthy addiction.

Unfortunately, it is not a great way to lose weight. There is calorie inflation on all the exercise equipment you are using. To sell treadmills, the calories being burned per hour are often exaggerated. One piece of cake will take a long time to burn off on a treadmill. However, for some people, starting an exercise program along with a diet is just the ticket. Their exercise regimen organizes their eating patterns and they eat fewer calories. If you restrict your exercise to set periods of exercising on a treadmill or a bicycle, you may compensate for this set exercise by being less active other times of the day. To prevent this, emphasize overall activity and include physical activity such as gardening, walking, using stairs, and so on. In this book you have learned how to exercise to maximize your results by building muscle to increase the number of calories you are burning, and walking or running to train your heart and reduce your stress. You have also learned how to use a pedometer to monitor your overall activity.

Myth #7
You Get All the Vitamins and Minerals You Need by Eating the Basic Four Food Groups

The basic four food groups were developed so that key nutrients such as calcium would be included in the diet. The idea was that by eating dairy foods you would get your calcium, and by eating red meat you would get your iron. Fruits and vegetables would give you your vitamin C, and breads, cereals, and grains would give you your fiber and other key vitamins. Foods were fortified with vitamin D, leading to the disappearance of rickets, a bone disease that resulted in bowed legs, commonly found in those born before the 1950s. Along the line, we drifted away from this idealized dietary pattern. Americans eat three servings a day of fruits and vegetables, and if their one fruit is ketchup and their vegetables are iceberg lettuce and French fries, they are missing the vitamins and minerals found in the many different-colored fruits and vegetables. A great deal of research demonstrates that while you should try to get your vitamins and minerals from your diet first, it is a good idea to take a multivitamin/multimineral every day to back up your best efforts. Vitamin C, vitamin E, and calcium round out my basic four vitamins and minerals to complement the basic four food groups.

Myth #8
Carrots and Bananas Are Fattening

Carrots and bananas were singled out in the Zone Diet as being fattening. Many of my patients who read or heard about that book remembered this myth. In fact, carrots are no more fattening than any vegetable in their class. They do contain sugar, but the amounts are small and come into play only when you make carrot juice, thus using large quantities of carrots. If you remove the fiber from carrots, it becomes possible to drink juice containing the sugar from ten carrots in a single glass of juice, adding up to 250 calories to your diet. Similarly, while the banana has no particular phytochemicals to warrant its inclusion in your diet every day, there are only about 100 calories in a small to medium banana. So adding a half banana to mixed fruit for taste is okay, but devouring three or four bananas, or, for that matter, overeating any fruit, can add significantly to your calories for the day.

Myth #9
Peanut Butter Is a Good Source of Protein

Peanuts are legumes, not nuts. They are high in fat, with about 80 percent of their calories coming from fat. The protein in nuts, like that in beans, is not a complete protein source due to the mix of amino acids found in nuts. In countries where nuts are the primary source of protein, the dietary patterns also tend to include plenty of fruits and vegetables. The context in which nuts are eaten is also relevant here. Nuts are a wonderful taste enhancer, and some nuts (such as almonds and walnuts eaten in amounts of about one ounce per day, or about eight nuts) provide a good source of monounsaturated fats, but a handful of nuts on the way to a double scotch and a prime rib are another matter altogether. Here the calories of the nuts are added to the rest of a high-fat meal and increase the risk of becoming overweight or obese.

Myth #10
Pork Is the Other White Meat

With the popularity of the white meat of chicken and turkey, the pork industry wanted to climb on the bandwagon and associate with winners. It is true that some cuts of pork can be as low in fat as chicken or turkey, but this does not apply to pork chops, pork sausage, and bacon. Nutrition experts uniformly classify pork as a red meat, and to say otherwise confuses consumers about the nature of white and red meats. Also, the dark meat of chicken and turkey is significantly higher in fat than the white meat, so it is not just chicken and turkey, but the white meat of chicken and turkey you should be selecting.

Myth #11
Eating More Margarine and
Vegetable Oils Lowers Cholesterol

This myth was based on work done in the 1950s at the Harvard School of Public Health. They found that if you use polyunsaturated vegetable oils or margarine instead of lard while matching total calories, then you will find that there is a lower cholesterol level in the individuals eating polyunsaturated fats and oils. These results cannot be translated into a public health recommendation because, in practice, adding fats to the diet, regardless of whether they are saturated or polyunsaturated, adds extra calories. Increases in the intake of vegetable oils were found at the same time as there was an increase in the incidence of obesity. Obesity increases cholesterol levels in most individuals who are susceptible to this effect (about one in four). And in the mid-1980s the Federal Trade Commission forced vegetable oil manufacturers to stop advertising the benefits of corn oil on cholesterol levels.

Myth #12
Eating Salmon Will
Lower Cholesterol Levels

Salmon is supposed to be a good source of healthy fish oils. However, it all depends on whether you are eating ocean-caught salmon or farmed salmon. The vast majority of salmon sold in this country comes from salmon farms. The most common is Atlantic salmon plopped into the Pacific Ocean in farms near Seattle, Washington. An eight-ounce slice of farmed salmon has twenty-one grams of fat, compared to only fourteen grams in ocean-caught salmon. The extra fat is not the healthy omega-3 fatty acid–enriched fish oils, but rather the omega-6 fatty acids from the grains and other feed these fish get from automated feeders. Unlike their counterparts in the ocean, which are athletic predators, these fish sit around all day growing in size as fast as they can. Trout and catfish are also farmed, so ask before buying these fish. Don't despair. There are lots of other healthy fish from the ocean, including halibut, swordfish, sea bass, whitefish, and sole.

Myth #13
Shrimp Will Raise Cholesterol Levels

Shrimp were once advertised as being high in cholesterol, but the picture has changed. The American Heart Association acknowledged a long time ago that shrimp had been wrongly accused, but lots of people, including some doctors, still believe this myth. Shrimp have about the same amount of cholesterol as the white meat of chicken. They are low in fat and calories and are a rich source of healthy omega-3 fatty acids. Most shrimp are grown in aquaculture farms and are pampered by being fed vegetable paste. If you can't be a vegetarian, eat a vegetarian shrimp. In studies where individuals are fed shrimp, a rise in blood cholesterol levels is not observed, since most cholesterol is made in the body by the liver rather than taken in from the diet.

Myth #14
Cheese Crackers Are a
Good Source of Calcium

Recently I saw an ad for cheese crackers that claimed they were now a good source of calcium. While food fortification with calcium can be beneficial, as in what has been done with orange juice, putting healthy nutrients into snack foods, which add more calories and fat to the diet without adding other nutrition, rubs me the wrong way. Instead of snacking on processed crackers, you could be eating fruits and vegetables and getting your calcium in either a supplement or in a healthy calcium-fortified food such as orange juice, tomato juice, or soy protein. The point is not to make jelly beans a vehicle for bringing healthy nutrition into your diet. This just generates confusion. Eat snacks such as these when you are not eating healthy, which should be less than 10 percent of the time.

Myth #15
Frozen Vegetables Aren't
as Good as Fresh

Some people think that freezing and thawing destroys so much in the way of vitamins that frozen vegetables aren't as good as fresh. This is not true. Fruits and vegetables frozen just after harvesting are picked when very ripe and tend to have more vitamins and phytonutrients than fruits and vegetables picked before ripening, while they are still hard. Frozen broccoli is a great source of the phytochemicals found in fresh broccoli. Tomatoes sent to market while still green are sprayed with ethylene gas to turn them red. Genetic research on the tomato has enabled the identification of the ripening gene, so that tomatoes that are rich in phytochemicals but also have a long shelf life have been developed. Freezing is a practical tool for getting vegetables distributed to places where they may not be grown naturally. Learning more about the genetics of plants and using standard breeding methods can improve the quality of our plant-based foods. So don't assume so-called natural is always better.

In the next section of this book, you will learn how the recommendations made above can help you reduce your risk of getting the most common and damaging diseases in our society, including heart disease, many common forms of cancer, and certain other diseases of aging. Not only does healthy nutrition put more years in your life, but it also helps to put more life in your years by improving your mental, physical, and sexual vitality.

COLORIZE FOR OPTIMUM WELLNESS

How DNA Damage Leads to Disease

o ahead, take a deep breath! You just inhaled a potentially toxic chemical that could seriously damage your DNA. I am not talking about smog or pollutants or cigarette smoke. We will get to those later! I am talking about the life-giving element in the air you breathe—oxygen. Oxygen makes up 20 percent of this air. The other 80 percent is made up mostly of nitrogen, with less than 1 percent as carbon dioxide. If I force you to breathe 100 percent oxygen, you will, over a period of days, go blind and suffer permanent damage to your lung tissue as a direct result of tissue damage caused by oxygen.

About twenty years ago oxygen poisoning of patients actually occurred in American hospitals' neonatal intensive care units, where premature babies were hooked up to 100 percent oxygen masks in an attempt to get adequate oxygen into their bloodstream and through their thickened and underdeveloped lungs. Ultimately, doctors discovered that vitamin E given to these babies could prevent a form of blindness (called "retrolental fibroplasia"). The vitamin E concentrated in the lung tissue and in other body tissues to counteract the effects of oxygen by trapping the extra electron on an oxygen radical—the chemically reactive harmful form of oxygen.

Your body can use oxygen in both positive and negative ways once it is absorbed. By the time you finish this chapter, you will understand how oxygen can be both the major life-giving element in our atmosphere and at the same time hold the key to the process of aging, the development of heart disease and cancer, and even the degeneration of mental function in Alzheimer's disease and other diseases of the brain.

In the first part of this book, you learned what to eat to protect your DNA. In this part you will learn *why*, and at the same time you will learn more about *how* to protect your DNA. If you have certain common diseases in your family, such as heart disease, diabetes, or cancer, you will learn much more about how damage to your DNA can cause these diseases to develop and how diet and lifestyle can prevent or delay their onset.

Common Diseases Have Common Causes

Common diseases occur commonly and many of them result from the imbalance of our genes and our modern diets and lifestyle. At the root of this gene-nutrient imbalance is the common occurrence of overactive defense mechanisms producing oxygen radicals that cannot be balanced by our antioxidant defense mechanisms. The best scientific evidence today points to oxygen radicals as the root stimulus for the development of heart disease, cancer, dementia, and premature aging.

Obviously, some diseases are so strongly determined by genes that nothing will deter their course or stop their development. Luckily, these are rare diseases that developed in special ways, which you will learn about. For such common diseases as diabetes, heart disease, and common forms of cancer, you will learn in the next few chapters that diet can delay, reduce the severity of, or prevent altogether many of them. All in all, I believe that you will be shocked to see how important your diet is to your overall health and longevity.

Oxygen Radicals Lead to
Damaged Cells, Dead Cells, and Cancer

As oxygen is drawn into your lungs with every breath you take, it is mixed into a fluid that lines the surface of your lungs. Remarkably, the surface area of your lungs is as large as a tennis court. Imagine spread over this tennis court a thin layer of fluid that contains vitamin C, vitamin E, and other antioxidants made in your body and derived from your diet. An oxygen molecule is made up of two oxygen atoms. These two atoms can break apart under the influence of heat or light. When this happens, you have two oxygen radicals that are simply oxygen atoms, each with an unpaired electron. This extra electron is like a spark in a gas tank—it can cause tiny atomic explosions that damage all the different parts of your cells, including the fat, the protein, and the DNA.

As long as there are enough protective antioxidants in the fluid to absorb the tiny explosions, your tissues won't be damaged. However, if you run out of or burn up these defenses by being exposed to smoke or other toxins, your lung cells will be damaged.

What is so bad about cell damage? Excessive damage to the DNA in your lung cells will cause them to die, and the immune system will simply clean up the dead cells. Minimal damage to the DNA can be repaired without noticeable damage to your cells. However, between these two extremes there is a level of damage that cannot be cleaned up and does not kill the cell. If the damage occurs in sensitive parts of the DNA, a lung cancer will develop.

Smoking Produces Oxygen Radicals and Eats Up Antioxidants

Smokers conduct an experiment on their lungs every day by depleting the protective substances around their lung cells. As they smoke they inactivate the protective antioxidants in the fluid bathing their lung cells. By rolling the dice every day that they smoke, they take the chance that just the right amount of damage to their DNA will occur to cause lung cancer. In fact, 85 percent of all lung cancer occurs in smokers. Smoking also promotes our number one killer disease—heart disease. You have probably heard so much about cholesterol, you may not realize that smoking promotes heart disease by using the same kinds of signals between cells that cause cancer.

If you want somebody to say something good about smoking, you've got the wrong book. While tobacco helped to establish this country, and slavery, back in the 1600s, it remains a killer drug that we export around the world. Classic films, where tobacco manufacturers paid to have

cigarettes smoked by leading men and their leading ladies, glamorized
the habit. In the 1940s one brand was called the "doctor's cigarette."
One out of every ten smokers will get lung cancer. And untold numbers
of heart attacks occur each year without anyone ascribing them to smoking. Many more will end up with lung diseases, and others will increase
their risk of ovarian cancer, stomach cancer, prostate cancer, and uterine
cancer. Cigars have become the luxury smoke of the new millennium and
those ten-dollar-and-up cigars have a whole pack's worth of nicotine and
tar in one cigar. Pipes and cigars lead to lip, tongue, and mouth cancer as
they eat up the defenses against oxygen damage to DNA right at the tissues first contacted by the air you are breathing.

Pollution and Oxygen Damage to DNA

You can damage DNA in a cell by using radiation or a poisonous chemical such as those used in chemotherapy for cancers. At high doses these
poisons kill the cell by activating oxygen radicals. Every day we are
taking in oxygen that has the potential to do the same type of harm to
our DNA at a lesser but more dangerous level. Our foods also contain
tiny amounts of chemicals that can damage DNA. We all live in a big
terrarium called Earth, and we have to drink and eat here on this earth,
not in some mystical pollution-free place. In fact, there are natural
carcinogens in the plants we eat that plants developed as a defense
against attacking insects. Luckily, the preventive substances in plants are
there in much greater quantity than the natural cancer-causing chemicals.
So you can't avoid cancer-causing chemicals, just as you cannot avoid
breathing in oxygen. You can eat the foods from the Color Code and
assure that you will get enough protective substances to reduce the
chance that DNA damage will lead to heart disease, cancer, or other common diseases.

There is some good news at the end of this scary story. Your body has
developed, at every level, great defense mechanisms against these pollutants and naturally occurring carcinogens. At the level of DNA, there are
repair mechanisms that can remove damaged DNA and replace that
DNA with what should be there. There are also systems of coordinated
defenses called the "antioxidant defense system." This is made up of proteins called "enzymes" that directly render oxygen radicals harmless or
else increase the levels of the antioxidant chemicals that do the same

thing. These systems evolved at a time when man was eating a diet rich in plant foods that provided antioxidants and other colorful preventive chemicals in the diet. In the last few hundred years, as we have narrowed the variety of the foods we eat, we have lost these compounds that the body was expecting to help defend the DNA.

The body uses oxygen radicals as part of the system to excrete toxins and drugs from the body. There is a two-step process in the liver and other tissues in which the electron on the oxygen radical is transferred to a toxic compound, making it able to react with another chemical that can dissolve in water (such as a sugar or a sulfur compound). When the activated compound and the sugar combine, the poison is no longer active and can be excreted from the body in your urine.

The chemicals in fruits, vegetables, and other plant foods trigger a number of protective reactions in your cells that defend your DNA from natural and artificial pollutants, and prevent most of the chronic diseases you will read about.

Why Is DNA Damage So Deadly?

DNA is the code of life, and its integrity is critical to every cell in your body. Mistakes happen in the duplication of the DNA code when a cell divides, and most of these happen in parts of the 90 percent of DNA that is not used to make proteins. This mysterious 90 percent somehow regulates the function of the remaining 10 percent. We know from the human genome project that this part of the DNA has many sequences repeated over and over again. If the DNA repair mechanisms are intact, many times an attack by an oxygen radical on DNA can be harmless. Some of these harmless changes, called "mutations," are kept in the DNA of the cell as it replicates itself. Sometimes, though, accumulated DNA damage can pile up until it reaches a critical level and cell damage results. If the cell dies, it can be removed by various cells of the immune system.

However, there are some changes in DNA that lead to the formation of a cancer cell. Cancer cells fight off the immune system and refuse to be cleared from the body. They put out proteins that help them grow their own blood supply. They don't respect the local boundaries in tissues and organs and, ultimately, they kill you. For the full story on cancer see chapter 12. Heart disease results first from oxygen damage to cholesterol, which enables cholesterol to stay in the walls of your blood vessels for a longer period of time. As it sits there, immune cells come and gobble up the oxygen-damaged cholesterol. Then the signals put out by these immune cells stimulate overgrowth of smooth muscle cells. The signals are similar to those made by cancer cells. In fact, while the signals put out by immune cells protect you from infections, this process can also be harmful and can stimulate cell growth, as in atherosclerosis in the heart, and in tumor cells. Sometimes infections are associated with both heart disease and cancer. In the stomach a bacteria called *Helicobacter pylori* can screw itself like a corkscrew into the lining of your stomach, setting up a lifelong infection. Immune cells try in vain to clear the bacteria. They try to kill it by using oxygen radicals and related chemicals. These oxygen radicals don't kill the bacteria; instead, they set up a chronic inflammation of the stomach lining called "atrophic gastritis." Then, after a few decades, stomach cancers develop in these areas. The good news is that in individuals who eat green and yellow vegetables in large amounts, the risk of this form of cancer is lower.

This is another illustration of how the Color Code of fruits and vegetables works to protect your DNA and prevent a serious life-threatening disease. Bacteria have been found in other surprising places as well. Evidence of infection with chlamydia bacteria has been found in blood vessel walls, and it has been proposed that the inflammation around these bacteria contribute to the progression of heart disease. For the full story on how genes and diet interact in heart disease see chapter 11.

The Antioxidant Defense System

Since oxygen has been around all living cells, from those in bacteria to those in chimpanzees, since the dawn of evolution, our bodies have a well-developed multitiered defense system against oxygen damage to DNA.

First, there are stored antioxidant chemicals that come from fruits and vegetables, herbs, teas, or dietary supplement pills. They can be stored in the body, as is the case with lycopene, lutein, and beta-carotene, or they can be broken down by the body extensively, as is the case with soy protein and green tea. This first system is dependent on diet, since many of these compounds, such as vitamin C, vitamin E, and lycopene, are not made in the body.

Second, the presence of these chemicals in the body triggers the genes in the liver and other tissues to develop proteins to break down the chemicals consumed in the diet in large amounts. This system is also dependent on the diet, since the liver of someone who takes in 500 milligrams per day of vitamin C will have developed the proteins needed to break down this vitamin C, while someone who eats no vitamin C at all will not have these same proteins in the liver. These proteins can sometimes also break down other substances from the environment that are similar in chemical structure to vitamin C, so the triggering of this genetic response to vitamin C may be helpful in warding off other potential cancer-causing chemicals.

Third, there is a well-developed DNA repair system that cuts out any damaged DNA and replaces it with the correct sequence of bases so that no damage will be apparent when the cell attempts to use the once damaged string of DNA. Substances in fruits and vegetables called "flavonoids" have been shown to activate the DNA repair system. So all the multitiered defenses we have against oxygen-radical damage depend critically on getting adequate protective substances from the diet.

Our antioxidant defense system evolved in a plant-based environment where many antioxidants could be obtained from the food supply. As a result, the genetic machinery to produce vitamin C was lost in humans, but our bodies came to expect a large amount of vitamin C and other plant chemicals in the diet. So we make some antioxidants and take others into our bodies from the food supply.

The Common Thread of Inflammation

The response of the immune cells in the body to an invading virus, bacterium, or tumor cell is similar. The immune defenses attack the invader directly with oxygen-radical production, or by releasing protein signals from cells that trigger oxygen damage. Just as your laundry bleach can kill bacteria and viruses, the natural bleach produced within cells in the form of oxygen radicals and related substances, such as hydrogen peroxide (found in bleach) and nitric oxide (made by the body), help the immune system rid your body of invaders.

Sometimes, there is a false alarm and these mechanisms are activated in error. The body sometimes interprets an insult such as smoking tobacco or eating a diet with too much fat and too many calories as if it were an invading organism. The process set up as a result of this false alarm is called "inflammation," and can damage your DNA.

Inflammation is common in many tissues, such as in the lungs of smokers, in the breast tissue of women eating a high-fat diet, and in the prostate tissues of men who have mild infections of the prostate gland (called "prostatitis"). Our natural defenses and those we obtain from our diets can neutralize some inflammation. However, when the diet is poor in antioxidants and rich in substances such as the fatty acids in corn oil that stimulate oxygen-radical formation, chronic inflammation sets up housekeeping and ultimately can lead to the type of DNA damage that promotes cancer and heart disease.

Diet and Inflammation: Hints from Aspirin

For many years we have known that taking aspirin, a simple over-the-counter medication, could reduce your risk of heart attacks and common forms of cancer such as colon cancer. Surveys show that men using aspirin daily have fewer heart attacks and are less likely to get colon cancer. The fact that aspirin works to prevent these diseases is directly related to the missing protective substances in our modern diets.

Aspirin is acetylsalicylic acid and comes from willow tree bark. It is also found in trace amounts in plant foods. In fact, our ancient diet was rich in substances similar to aspirin that counteracted inflammation, while our modern diet is full of things that promote inflammation, such as the polyunsaturated fats found in corn oil and other vegetable oils.

While all dietary fats, from lard to safflower oil, have the same calorie content (140 calories per tablespoon), there are many variations in the molecular structure of fats. The most basic structural components of fats are the *fatty acids*. These are classified by chemical names based on their structure and properties.

Saturated fatty acids are solid at room temperature and predominate in lard and butter. Monounsaturated fatty acids (so named because they have one double bond between carbons in the fatty acid molecule) predominate in avocados and olives, and are liquid at room temperature. Polyunsaturated fats are also liquid at room temperature and have more than one double bond (three to six such bonds are found in the most common fatty acids).

Polyunsaturated fatty acids come in two main classes, omega-3 and omega-6, named according to where the first double bond occurs on the carbon chain. Human beings evolved on a diet comprised of about equal amounts of omega-3 and omega-6 fatty acids—a ratio of about one to one, found in fruits, vegetables, and other plant foods. Over the past century there has been an enormous increase in the quantity of omega-6 fats in the human diet. The source of this increase has been vegetable oils processed from corn, sunflower seeds, safflower seeds, cottonseed, and soybeans. These oils are common ingredients in processed foods such as chips, breads, cookies, and soft ice creams, and are often used for cooking. Today, in typical Western diets, the ratio of omega-6 to omega-3 fatty acids ranges from twenty to one to thirty to one.

Because the human genome evolved to suit a very different ratio of fatty acids than the Western diet offers, high omega-6 intake causes a physiologic shift that can adversely affect health in many ways. According to nature's design, fats are consumed in small amounts as part of whole foods. When oils are extracted from grains or nuts and added in large quantities to other foods, they are bound to cause imbalances. Those imbalances can have significant effects on human biology.

Meat eaten until the dawn of modern livestock farming came from animals that fed on grasses, while today's meats are from animals fed mostly on grains. Fats found in the flesh of grass-fed animals contain more omega-3s than those found in the flesh of modern livestock raised on a steady diet of grain. The fat of grain-fed animals is richer in omega-6s.

Overconsumption of omega-6s changes the balance of specialized hormones called "prostaglandins." A high intake of these fats as vegetable oils and animal foods promotes the formation of these prostaglandins, which precipitate heart attacks and out-of-control inflammation. (Allergies, asthma, eczema, and rheumatoid arthritis are also examples of inflammation run amok.) One type of omega-6 fatty acid, linoleic acid, has been found, in laboratory studies, to stimulate the growth of prostate cancer cells and to promote the growth and spread of breast cancer in mice and rats.

Linoleic acid acts not just as a nutrient, but can also cause changes in the functioning of cells by binding to a protein called the "PPAR-gamma" (peroxisome proliferator activating receptor-gamma). This protein binds to one of the prostaglandins (PGJ3) made from linoleic acid. This PPAR-gamma receptor is found in tumor cells, where it may be responsible for some of the effects of omega-6 fatty acids on tumor growth. It is also present in the white cells in the walls of the heart's blood vessels, where it may contribute to the process of atherosclerosis. What we have in linoleic acid is an example of a fatty acid that acts both as a nutrient and as a signal for cellular actions in the body.

Vegetable oils such as corn oil, sunflower oil, safflower oil, and soybean oil are extremely rich in linoleic acid. They contain eight to ten times more linoleic acid than monounsaturated oils (olive and avocado oil). Canola oil has about three times as much linoleic acid as olive oil. None of these oils is rich in the omega-3 fatty acids.

Monounsaturated fatty acids, found most abundantly in olive and avocado oils, don't tip the balance of the specialized hormones one way or the other. They do, however, have calories and many of the taste-enhancing effects of fats and oils. If the calories don't matter, extra-virgin olive oil or avocado oil can lower cholesterol when substituted calorie for calorie for the saturated fat found in a prime rib. However, be aware that if you gain weight, your cholesterol will go up.

The mixture of fatty acids stored in your fat tissue is a reflection of the kinds of fatty acids you've eaten over the past year. If you've overdone it with the omega-6s and saturated fats, your fat stores will be high in linoleic acid. When I place patients on a very low fat diet, the levels of linoleic acid in their blood and tissue fluids fall by 30 percent. Such a large shift can positively affect blood clotting, blood-fat levels, immune function, and inflammation throughout the body.

A sizable body of research has shown that adding omega-3 fatty acids to the diet helps to prevent coronary artery disease, high blood pressure, and type 2 diabetes. Omega-3s are also proving to be a useful therapy for kidney disease, rheumatoid arthritis, ulcerative colitis, Crohn's disease, and some types of lung disease.

Most of the studies performed to prove the usefulness of supplemental omega-3 fatty acids used fish oils. While omega-3 fatty acids are found in some vegetable oils, the body is relatively inefficient in converting the shorter eighteen carbon-length fatty acids, such as those found in flaxseed, into the active twenty and twenty-two carbon-length fatty acids that are called "fish oil fatty acids" (EPA and DHA, or eicosapentanoic acid and docosahexanoic acid).

How Fruits and Vegetables
Protect Your DNA

Fruits and vegetables protect your DNA by counteracting the inflammation process described above. By eating a diet based on fruits and vegetables, you will have lowered your dietary intake of total fats and polyunsaturated fats as well as refined sugars. You will also have increased your intake of antioxidants and anti-inflammatory protective substances from the diverse colored fruits and vegetables you are now eating. In the next few chapters you will learn that these common threads of inflammation and oxidation, which cause diseases in the absence of a healthy diet, are only the beginning. In many ways, your body has been designed for the type of plant-rich diet based on the Color Code. The imbalance between our diet, evolved over the last few hundred years, and our genes, which evolved over the last 100,000 years, causes profound dislocations in the machinery of many cells throughout our bodies. In the next chapter you will see how overweight and obesity, the most common nutritional disorders in our society, increase inflammation as well. Then you will learn how the Color Code can reduce your risk of heart disease, common forms of cancer, Alzheimer's disease, and accelerated aging.

10

The Surprising Fat Cell: Much More Than a Bag of Fat

You probably think your fat cells are simply a place to store fat, but you would probably be surprised to find out that they play a number of key roles in your body, including:

- Secreting inflammatory hormones called "cytokines" that protect you against infections but which in excess promote inflammation, blood clotting, and chronic diseases, including heart disease and common forms of cancer.
- Acting like a hormone gland to convert male hormones into female hormones.
- Storing protective antioxidants, including vitamin E and many of the colored chemicals in fruits and vegetables.
- Storing calories efficiently so that you can survive for prolonged periods of time without food.
- Storing fatty acids that you eat and those you make from carbohydrates and proteins, so that in terms of the balance of pro-inflammatory and anti-inflammatory fatty acids in your fat cells, you are what you eat.

Fat Cells Act Like White Blood Cells

Fat cells secrete hormones and pro-inflammatory substances, called "cytokines," that are part of the immune system defenses usually associated with your white blood cells. Cytokines play a key role in the defense against infection, just as they play a key role in the defense against starvation.

Leptin, the fat-cell hormone, is a cytokine. Leptin was first discovered in an inbred strain of obese mice that were identical to normal mice, with the exception of a mutation in a gene for one protein. The gene was known to be defective, because if the blood circulation of a thin mouse was hooked up to one of these obese mice, the fat mouse would become thin. After several decades of mouse breeding, modern genetic technology enabled researchers at Rockefeller University, led by Dr. Jeff Friedman and Dr. Rudy Leibel, to isolate the protein, which they named "leptin," from the Greek word for "thinning."

The Best-Laid Plans of Mice and Men

After the discovery of leptin, the hormone was made in the laboratory and given as an injection to obese mice that were made fat not by genetics but by eating what is called a "cafeteria diet." Most mice and rats are fed pretty tasteless pellets, made from grains and refined sugar with vitamins and minerals added, called "chow." This looks a lot like dog chow, and if you have had a picky-eating pet, you know that you sometimes have to dress up this chow to make it appealing. When scientists put chocolate chip cookies, peanut butter, and high-fat meats in the chow, mice go to town. They eat so much that they get as fat as the genetically obese mice.

When scientists injected leptin into the overfed mice eating the cafeteria diet, they, too, became thin. Leptin acts on the appetite center of the brain to reduce the drive to eat, and in mice it increases physical activity. This was enough evidence for Amgen, a biotech pharmaceutical company in Thousand Oaks, California, to plop down $20 million for an exclusive license to develop leptin as a cure for obesity.

Is Leptin the Cure for Fat?

Studies with leptin are still proceeding, but the results so far indicate that humans are resistant to the effects of leptin at the doses achievable by injection, and show only a statistically detectable but small weight loss. However, the amount of leptin in the blood is directly proportional to the percent of body fat in men and women. We still don't fully understand leptin regulation, but it is secreted in pulses throughout the day and night with the lowest levels occuring at night, while you are not eating.

Leptin Is Part of the Immune System

There are a few families in Turkey with an inborn leptin deficiency. They die prematurely of infections, so the functions of leptin may be to protect you against malnutrition and the infections associated with malnutrition. Leptin and other cytokines are secreted from fat cells, and the ability to form fat cells is a favorable trait in societies where malnutrition and infectious diseases are common.

However, when you overeat and accumulate excess fat cells, as in our modern society in the United States, your fat cells put out increased levels of a number of cytokines, including leptin, that increase the oxidative damage to your DNA and thus promote heart disease and common forms of cancer. So the immune system, developed like our energy storage system for times of famine, cannot cope with excess calories and fat without stimulating harmful inflammation and oxidation.

Fat Cells Store Colorful Chemical Protectors

Fat cells also store many of the colored chemicals found in fruits and vegetables and release these, together with fat, into the bloodstream. They store antioxidants such as vitamin E as well, so they hold the key to counteracting some of the many pesticides and toxins in the environment that are also stored in fat.

If someone drinks large amounts of carrot juice, their skin will turn bright orange. While I am not advocating that you do this, it does illustrate how the fat under the skin and throughout the body can store fat-soluble antioxidants such as the beta-carotene and alpha-carotene in carrots.

Fat Cells, Fat Cells—Everywhere

Fat cells are everywhere. They are under your skin, where they determine if you have the soft contours of a woman or the hard body of a man. They are in your liver, where they influence the storage and production of fats that circulate in your bloodstream. They are in your muscle, where they affect the amount of carbohydrate versus fat energy being burned during exercise and the effectiveness of insulin in driving sugar into your muscles.

Fat cells are a key organ in the body, just like the kidney or the liver. There is a way to genetically engineer mice so that their fat cells never mature to carry out their normal functions. Those animals become diabetic because they cannot store energy as fat. Their blood sugar levels go sky-high. Fat may not be something you like looking at, but your fat plays many important roles in keeping your body healthy.

How Many Fat Cells Do You Need?

The human body contains billions of fat cells. Many years ago there was a theory based on studies on rats and mice that you had all your fat cells in place before puberty and that they just got bigger after puberty. This theory suggested that if you developed too many fat cells as a child, you were doomed to be fat all your life as your fat cells got bigger without going away. Luckily, this theory is not correct. In fact, your body can recruit an infinite number of fat cells throughout life whenever you need to store more fat.

Fat Cells That Won't Go Away

Some fat cells put in place by sex hormones or overnutrition, especially under the skin (so-called subcutaneous fat), may be resistant to your weight-reduction efforts that incorporate diet and exercise. These cells can sometimes be removed by liposuction, but you better be careful.

While the cells that are removed never come back, cells all around the area can grow back, giving you an ugly dimpled look. If you are considering liposuction as a cosmetic procedure, be sure your diet is under great control for at least one or two years before proceeding.

More important than these localized pockets of fat, women should realize that their body-fat distribution changes throughout life. With your first child, the body's fat moves around. It usually goes to the hips and thighs, but some women also gain weight in the upper body. You should always aim to get your body fat down to a healthy level, but don't be unrealistic. You cannot turn the clock back to your teens when you are in your forties or fifties. Your fat cells just won't cooperate.

Fat distribution into pockets and lumps is also determined genetically. With identical twins, not only is the amount of fat in the bodies similar, but the distribution of the fat in different parts of the body is virtually identical. We don't know why exactly, but fat is deposited in different places in each individual to carry out its essential functions.

Fat Cells Are Serious Business

Are fat cells just a cosmetic pain in the neck? Were they put on earth to make you miserable? Actually, fat cells are part of the immune system that protects your body from infectious diseases.

In the middle of the Pacific, there is a small island that was inhabited for thousands of years by a stable population of about three thousand individuals. In the 1800s a group of European explorers arrived on the island and immediately infected the population with a virus that was deadly to it. About 90 percent of the island's population was wiped out. The three hundred remaining individuals gave birth to succeeding generations in which obesity was the normal state. Why were the genetics for hanging on to fat important to the remaining three hundred islanders? Very simply, avoiding malnutrition provided them with the ability to survive the infectious onslaught by maintaining their immune function. How are they doing now? They have a high incidence of high blood pressure, diabetes, and gout.

This same scenario of infectious disease setting the table for development of obesity was played out across Europe in the Middle Ages, so the tendency toward obesity may have something to do with mankind's past exposure to infectious diseases.

Small Babies Sometimes
Make Fat Grown-ups

Your brain, including the center regulating appetite, has not yet fully developed when you are still in your mother's womb. Studies of babies who were small in the womb show that they are more likely to be obese as teenagers. These babies eat voraciously after they are born, whether from the bottle or the breast, until they make up for much of their under-weight and slow growth while in the uterus. When this malnutrition in the womb was studied in mice, the brain centers for feeding were found to have high levels of hormones promoting overeating right after birth, logically explaining this phenomenon.

Humans Are Well-Adapted
to Starvation, Not Overnutrition

When malnourished while in the uterus, the babies' levels of leptin fall, permitting another hormone, called "NPY," to rise. NPY is the feeding hormone, just as leptin is the thinning hormone. While in the uterus, the baby cannot get any more calories even with a high NPY, because the mother, for one reason or another, cannot deliver more calories to it. She is either severely malnourished herself, which will reduce the size of the baby, or has smoked cigarettes or otherwise damaged the circulation to the baby (through an organ in the uterus called the "placenta"). However, once the baby is born, the high NPY levels lead to increased feeding activity. As the baby gains body fat, the leptin levels rise along with the rise in body fat, but the NPY levels don't fall, so the baby keeps gaining weight. Obese adults also have high leptin levels proportionate to their increased body fat, but for some reason many keep overeating. The likely reason is that the feeding center's NPY does not fall appropriately in the obese adult either. From an evolutionary point of view, this all makes sense. When you are malnourished, you are driven to eat more. However, just because you found some food today, that doesn't mean you will have an endless supply. So nature doesn't worry about efficiently turning off the storage of fat, which then leads to obesity.

Fat Can Make You Sexy

The Good Book says "be fruitful and multiply." Increasing body fat increases the levels of sex hormones circulating in the body, and ultimately leads to increased fertility. In Egypt, after agriculture was discovered, the Hebrews were given fertile land in Goshen where they multiplied to such numbers as to threaten the pharoah. Well, you know the rest of the story. Among the adaptations to starvation is a decrease in sex drive and fertility in most women, although some are still fertile even in the face of food shortages. Men tend to retain their fertility with starvation, just as they do into old age. In fact, a man needs only 1 million functioning sperm, from a usual average of 100 million, to be fertile.

Fat Can Keep You Fertile

The *Venus of Willendorf* is a statue of a woman who lived some 24,000 years ago and shared with many fertility goddesses of that time a body type that most today would consider overweight. Her body fat is in the upper body, in a large abdomen and large, pendulous breasts, and she has relatively muscular legs supporting her upper-body weight. These were the desirable women of ancient times. They were more likely to bear healthy children, and they were able to suckle them when other women became infertile and unable to breast-feed.

Ancient Advantage
Becomes Modern Disease

Today about 5 percent of all women have a "disease" called polycystic ovarian syndrome, or PCO. It used to be called Stein-Leventhal syndrome after two doctors who rediscovered this ancient adaptation to starvation. All they knew was that many women were complaining to them about irregular periods, obesity, and excess body and facial hair.

When these women lose weight, their periods become regular and they become fertile. In some cases, their excess hair growth is reduced. These women have a form of type 2 diabetes of the ovary. The ovary has leptin and insulin receptors, and these women have very high insulin levels that push their ovaries to make more male hormones. As a result, they have more muscle than average women, and they tend to accumulate their body fat in a male pattern, in the upper body. A drug called "metformin" (Glucophage is the trade name) that corrects some of the insensitivity to insulin in type 2 diabetes has been shown to help these women as well. I often tell such women that they have great genes in the "wrong" century. They were the most desired of women in ancient times, due to their ability to remain fertile, and to perform physcial work even when food was in scarce supply. In recent years, we have valued thinness in women over these other traits. The thin Twiggy-like women models would probably have been starving under the conditions of ancient times and would have suffered infertility and chronic infections.

How Much Body Fat Is the Right Amount?

We each have a programmed amount of body fat that would perfectly balance our genes with our environment. I haven't lost any patients yet to fat deficiency, because there is enough healthy fat within fruits and vegetables and whole grains to provide more than the 5 percent of total calories needed in the diet as the essential plant fatty acids (linoleic and linolenic acids). In general, a total of 15 to 20 percent body fat for men and 22 to 28 percent body fat for women is ideal. Less than this ratio occurs in athletes who have increased muscle mass, and you may have to settle for more if you have lost muscle with aging. Whatever the amount of fat you have, in this range or higher, you will have enough fat to carry out its beneficial functions of storing healthy fatty acids, colored chemicals, and antioxidant vitamins, and protecting your body from infections by secreting cytokines. By reducing your excess body fat, especially in the upper body, you will be decreasing your risk of common chronic diseases.

How the Color Code Helps

If you have excess body fat, the Color Code, along with the individualization of protein and calories, is the simplest thing you can do to lose your excess fat while improving your health. The Color Code will reduce your total calories in a healthy way.

The benefits of the Color Code were recently demonstrated in a town in Finland where people were commonly dying of heart disease. The inhabitants told the mayor of this town, North Karelia, that he had to do something. A plan was devised that included the use of bike paths and other incentives to healthy living. In terms of diet, there was one simple strategy—increase fruit and vegetable intake. Whenever someone in the town ordered food at a restaurant, they paid for the entrée, but all the fruits and vegetables they could eat were free. Body weight, cholesterol, triglycerides, and other nutritional indicators all improved. So the Color Code is not only a great individual strategy, it is also a public health strategy.

In the next few chapters you will see how the Color Code is related to reducing the risk and severity of many common diseases.

11

Heart Disease, Cholesterol, and Your DNA

n the 1980s it seemed that polite cocktail conversation at southern California parties revolved around two numbers: property values and cholesterol counts. The "in crowd" was proud of the profits they were making in the soaring real estate market as their property values went up, while they were equally proud of their dropping cholesterol levels as they changed their diet and lifestyle.

Most of us have been taught that high cholesterol is the cause of heart attacks, but the cause-and-effect relationship doesn't always hold up. A professor at my university had a cholesterol count over 300 and lived without heart disease well into her eighties, while many seemingly fit individuals with so-called borderline high cholesterol (between 200 and 220) suffer heart attacks in their mid-fifties. Cholesterol is an important part of the big picture of heart disease, but it certainly doesn't tell the whole story. As is the case with most of the chronic diseases that tend to arise as we age, heart disease is almost always the result of an interaction between genes and diet.

The drug industry has been instrumental in spreading the word to doctors and patients about the relationship of high cholesterol levels to heart disease. It has profited greatly from these efforts because the drugs now used to lower cholesterol are expensive and widely prescribed.

Many of the advertisements for cholesterol-lowering drugs are misleading to the public because they oversimplify the cause-and-effect relationship between cholesterol and heart disease. You don't see actors in these ads portraying overweight couch potatoes eating greasy cheeseburgers in front of the television. They portray healthy people who embrace healthy lifestyles and still have high cholesterol, which gives the impression that the only solution for high cholesterol levels is drug therapy.

While these drugs have a place in the treatment of people who have already had a heart attack or who are in imminent danger of having one, they do so at great cost to our health care system. For prevention in the general population, there are far less expensive alternatives. Understanding those alternatives begins with an understanding of how gene-diet interaction can predispose you to high cholesterol and heart disease.

What Is Cholesterol?

Although cholesterol receives a great deal of attention in our heart attack–prone culture, not many people know exactly what this substance is or how it might increase heart disease risk. Cholesterol is a type of fat that is only made in the bodies of animals. While it can be made in almost any tissue, most of it is manufactured in the liver. Foods containing cholesterol are not the only source of this nutrient, because the liver makes as much as 75 percent of our cholesterol as long as it has sufficient raw materials to build it with. The manufacture of cholesterol and its transport from the liver to the rest of the body are under exquisite control. Cholesterol, a key molecule in so many body processes, is one of the most carefully regulated through control of both cholesterol production and excretion from the body.

Cholesterol has many uses in the body. It is the stuff from which the hormones cortisol, progesterone, testosterone, and estrogen are built. It is a structural component of the membranes of cells, and it is needed for the production of bone-building vitamin D.

Plants contain no cholesterol. Many plant foods (e.g., beans) contain chemicals called "phytosterols," which block the absorption of cholesterol in the gut. Today, foods containing phytosterols are recommended to reduce high blood cholesterol levels. Ancient humans, eating a low-cholesterol, plant-rich diet, however, had to find ways to conserve and maintain cholesterol so that their cells could get as much as they needed.

Not only did our ancestors eat little cholesterol, but the large amounts of plant foods they ate partly blocked its absorption. A diet rich in meats and dairy products but poor in fruits and vegetables, when combined with these genes is a prescription for high cholesterol.

Like other fats, cholesterol doesn't dissolve in the blood (which is water based), and must be carried in the circulation attached to proteins. There are two major types of protein carriers for cholesterol. One of these proteins, LDL (low-density lipoprotein), is designed to deposit cholesterol as it circulates. High-density lipoprotein, or HDL, picks up cholesterol as it travels through the vast network of blood vessels that feed every body cell and transports it back to the liver, where it is made into bile and then eliminated. Think of LDL as a cholesterol distributor, departing the liver with a full load and dumping it throughout the body, and think of HDL as a cholesterol eliminator, picking up the excess and taking it to the liver for disposal.

LDL cholesterol is easily oxidized. This means that it is subject to attack by free radicals, at which point it becomes a free radical itself and can cause damage to blood-vessel walls. This is one reason why it's so important to eat plenty of fresh vegetables and fruits, which naturally provide you with the antioxidants necessary to block oxidation.

HDL is more stable and doesn't oxidize easily. There is evidence that it is oxidized LDL cholesterol, since it is deposited in the artery wall more efficiently, not cholesterol itself, that contributes to the development of coronary artery disease.

If you haven't done so already, it's a good idea to have your cholesterol measured. The results of this fasting blood test will help you to recognize whether you have a genetic tendency toward high cholesterol; if so, you can change your diet before heart disease takes hold. Total cholesterol over 240 mg/dl (milligrams per deciliter of blood) may warrant treatment with medication; levels between 200 and 240 mg/dl can be remedied with diet and supplements. A better measurement of risk is your LDL count. If it is higher than 160 mg/dl, medication might be a good option, and if it falls between 130 and 160 mg/dl, diet and supplements should do the trick. HDL levels should be at least 50 mg/dl.

Most blood-chemistry tests will also measure triglycerides, another type of blood fat that can reflect increased heart disease risk if levels climb too high. Ideally, your triglycerides should be below 150 mg/dl.

If your cholesterol counts come back high, alter your diet for about two months using the guidelines in this book, and then have another blood test done to measure your cholesterol levels. If they haven't budged, taking a dietary supplement called Hong Qu, or red yeast rice (discussed in chapter 6), is an appropriate next step. Have another test done after two months on Hong Qu. If your numbers still haven't come down, your physician can give you a prescription for a cholesterol-lowering medication. Since all prescription drugs have side effects of some kind, it's always preferable to first try the simplest, most down-to-earth solutions such as diet and exercise.

The Making of a Heart Attack

Known in medical circles as "myocardial infarction," a heart attack is the result of a blockage in one or more of the blood vessels that carry oxygen-rich blood to the muscular walls of the heart. These vessels—the coronary arteries—wrap around the heart, twisting and turning to feed every part of this hard-working organ.

Many factors contribute to heart disease, including stress levels, blood pressure, homocysteine and triglyceride levels, and the tendency of the blood to clot. However, cholesterol is a major player in the process and an easily tested marker. Cholesterol, floating in the blood bound to LDL, can pass through the walls of the cells lining the coronary arteries. When oxidized cholesterol becomes trapped there, immune cells—white blood cells called "macrophages"—move into the area to engulf the oxidized cholesterol. These macrophages take up cholesterol as though they were gorging at a feast. Eventually they burst, releasing cholesterol into the space under the surface of the blood vessel.

This cholesterol, along with specific immune-cell signals, stimulates the growth of the cells lining the artery and draws more white blood cells into the area in an attempt to facilitate repair. An inflammatory bulge called a "plaque" develops inside the blood vessel. Plaques first become visible as yellow streaks in the lining of the coronary arteries. In American men who die in wars or in accidents while still in their early twenties, these changes can often already be seen in autopsies. Plaque buildup in the arteries is also known as atherosclerosis.

While it was once thought that cholesterol must completely block an artery to cause a heart attack, heart attacks usually happen when there is only about a 40 percent blockage in one or more coronary arteries. The deposit of cholesterol causing this partial blockage is unstable and breaks open, causing the formation of a clot. A heart attack occurs as the clot suddenly cuts off blood flow to an area of the heart muscle. Deprived of oxygen, that piece of the heart muscle either suffers permanent damage or dies. The important role of clot formation in heart attacks means that you should chew an aspirin while having chest pain. Aspirin, a product of the plant world derived from willow tree bark and other plants, makes the platelets forming the clot in your heart's artery less sticky. By taking aspirin during a heart attack, you will be partially blocking the clot formation that could result in a heart attack. Once the paramedics arrive, they can sometimes reduce the damage caused by a heart attack by infusing into your veins special enzymes that will break up clots.

Heart disease, still the number one killer of Americans, causes more than 700,000 deaths every year. Modern medical technology can unclog coronary arteries and keep heart attack patients alive if the problem is attended to quickly enough, but the heart is rarely left unscathed after a heart attack. Its pumping strength is usually compromised, and the risk of another heart attack continues to loom even after the ordeal is over.

Genes for High Cholesterol?

Cholesterol levels are very sensitive to a number of dietary influences, including calorie, fat, and fiber intake. I've seen cholesterol levels jump when patients of mine return from a cruise and too many midnight suppers. Both obesity and type 2 diabetes raise cholesterol levels. Some experts attribute the 20 percent tax-season rise in accountants' cholesterol levels to stress, but I think that Chinese-American take-out is an equally likely culprit.

For a small minority of those who end up with heart disease, a well-defined genetic flaw is to blame. This alteration in the genes causes what is known as type IIA hypercholesterolemia. The altered gene causes an abnormality in the proteins that carry cholesterol in the bloodstream, resulting in the deposit of excessive amounts of cholesterol into the walls of the coronary arteries.

There is very little cholesterol in a plant-based diet, and a number of natural substances inhibit the absorption and production of cholesterol. It's easy to see why genes conserving cholesterol were beneficial when foods containing it were scarce. Again, it's a case of great genes in the wrong environment. In light of the fact that almost one in four

Americans—a total of about 57 million—has coronary artery disease, however, it's obvious that there must be a variety of causes.

Cholesterol levels are carefully regulated in the body. The rate of production of cholesterol in a cell is reduced when the amount of cholesterol it contains increases. Certain strains of mice regulate cholesterol exquisitely and are resistant to coronary artery disease, while other strains don't suppress cholesterol synthesis as well and end up with heart disease on a high-cholesterol diet. This sort of genetic variation also appears in humans.

The Tarahumara Indians of northern Mexico are physically active, and eat, on average, only about 100 to 150 milligrams of cholesterol a day as part of a plant-based diet. Their blood-cholesterol levels are generally quite low—between 100 and 150 mg/dl, and heart disease, hypertension, and diabetes are unusual. Genetically similar members of the same tribe who live in southern Arizona and follow a Western diet eat an average of 300 to 800 milligrams of cholesterol a day, and their blood cholesterol levels are between 200 and 300 mg/dl. These people on the modern diet have among the highest rates of obesity and hypertension in the world. The genes of Tarahumara Indians are very well adapted to their highly active lifestyle in the mountains of northern Mexico. They cannot adapt to a diet of doughnuts, cakes, pastries, and foods with other fats and hidden sugars, and so their bodies gain fat and their cholesterol levels rise.

On the other side of the spectrum, the Masai in Africa consume a diet composed mostly of the meat, milk, and blood of cattle, and they have extremely low cholesterol levels. Among the Masai heart disease is virtually unheard of, and their cholesterol levels are low by comparison to the Tarahumaras. They have a very sensitive system for adjusting cholesterol production in the body in response to increased cholesterol intake.

I recently met a brilliant scientist at a conference and I invited him to my office, thinking I could help him improve his health. He was in his mid-thirties and overweight by forty or so pounds, and I had noticed at dinner during the conference that he indulged in high-fat meat and dessert. My plan was to help him lower his undoubtedly high cholesterol levels and shed some of the extra weight he carried around. After I had sat down with him and talked up the importance of maintaining healthy cholesterol levels, his lab results came back and showed his total cholesterol to be only 120 mg/dl! Some genetic endowment from his

Scandinavian heritage had geared his cells to downregulate cholesterol production quite efficiently when he ate high-cholesterol foods.

Statin Drugs and Red Yeast Rice

Statin drugs such as lovastatin are the most commonly prescribed medications for high cholesterol. They work by blocking an enzyme needed to make cholesterol in the body. They also act to stabilize cholesterol deposits in the blood-vessel wall, decreasing the likelihood that they will burst open and cause clots to form. While statin drugs can prevent heart attacks, they can cause some unpleasant side effects (muscle pain and liver damage) and are quite expensive, sometimes costing as much as several hundred dollars a month. These drugs are used by only some 5 million Americans among the 57 million with undesirably high levels of cholesterol. Fortunately, there is a natural substance that has the same beneficial effects and few of the liabilities of the statin drugs: a Chinese red yeast grown on rice, called Hong Qu, or red yeast rice, discussed in chapter 6. It is relatively inexpensive and safe, and is effective in lowering cholesterol levels.

At pennies per day, this yeast could decrease deaths from heart disease by 30 percent. I hope that someday Hong Qu will be a well-known, cost-effective nutritional supplement and alternative to statin drugs.

Other plant compounds that have cholesterol-lowering effects include the phytosterols (plant sterols), found in soy and other beans; substances known as limonoids, found in the oil of lemon and orange rinds; and tocotrienols, found in plant oils, such as a rice bran oil, that also contain vitamin E.

Apolipoprotein B

Once cholesterol has been made in a liver cell, it needs to be attached to a protein to move out of the cell. The protein that carries cholesterol out of the liver is called apolipoprotein B, or apo B for short. This protein becomes incorporated into LDL particles as cholesterol is released into the bloodstream. It has been found that the LDL of some individuals contains more apo B than others. Those with genes for making small, dense

LDL usually also have a high level of triglycerides and a low level of HDL. At least one large study has found that people with small, dense LDL have dramatically increased heart disease risk in comparison with those who have large LDL.

In ancient times, when dietary cholesterol was scarce, small, dense LDL was a good thing. The smaller particles can more easily pass through cell walls to deliver needed cholesterol to tissues. Now that humankind indulges in lots of high-fat, high-cholesterol foods, small, dense LDL has become a liability rather than an advantage. Some studies have shown that diet changes and exercise can increase the size of small, dense LDL and reduce heart disease risk. The more commonly prescribed cholesterol-lowering drugs—the statins—have no effect on increasing the size of these small, dense LDL particles. High-dose niacin, a B vitamin sometimes used to treat high cholesterol, can work to increase the size of small, dense LDL.

Lipoprotein(a)—Lp(a) for short—is a cholesterol-carrying protein much like LDL. While higher levels of this protein are associated with an increased risk of heart disease, some studies suggest that the risk is only present when total cholesterol and triglycerides are also high. Lp(a) levels are stable over the lifetime of each individual. They can vary up to a thousandfold between individuals, however, which shows us that Lp(a) levels are strongly determined by genes.

Floating on the surface of Lp(a) particles is another protein, apolipoprotein(a). Apo(a) is unique to Lp(a). Apo(a) is structurally similar to a molecule that promotes blood clotting. This effect of apo(a) carried on Lp(a) could explain the increase in heart disease risk with high Lp(a) levels.

There is still much we don't know about Lp(a). It's possible that it is a more important risk factor in some cases than in others, because different inherited forms of the protein have different effects on the clotting process. The B vitamin niacin, fish oils, and estrogen will sometimes lower Lp(a) levels, but don't do so consistently. If your blood work comes back showing elevations in this lipoprotein, let this motivate you to aggressively lower LDL cholesterol to 100 mg/dl or less. The risk of elevated Lp(a) is dependent on having elevated levels of cholesterol and triglycerides. If you have genetically elevated Lp(a), be sure your blood levels of cholesterol and triglycerides are well-controlled to reduce your risk of heart disease.

Very low density lipoproteins, called VLDL, primarily carry triglycerides but also contain about 20 percent of their lipids as cholesterol. VLDL also has a characteristic surface protein called apolipoprotein E (apo E). The gene that codes for apo E is polymorphic (has more than one expression), and each of the three common forms—apo E2, apo E3, and apo E4—reflects a different level of heart disease risk. Double copies of E4 and E2 (one copy from each parent) confer an increased risk of heart disease. In the chromosomes of 30 percent of Europeans, there is one copy of apo E4. Only 7 percent have two copies of apo E4, and 4 percent have two copies of apo E2. Eighty percent of Europeans have at least one copy of the E3 version of apo E; 39 percent have two copies. The farther north you travel in Europe, the more common apo E4 becomes. Three times more Swedes and Finns have apo E4 than Italians. Forty percent of African Americans, Polynesians, and Africans have the apo E4 polymorphism, while more than 50 percent of New Guineans have it. Asians have the lowest occurrence of E4 at about 15 percent.

Gene-nutrient interactions observed in these populations match what one might expect, knowing the effect of each version of apo E. Heart disease rates rise as one moves from southern to northern Europe, roughly in proportion to the frequency of apo E4 in the population. As long as New Guineans stick to their traditional diet of plants and lean bush meat, they don't have a particularly high incidence of heart disease, but if they shift to a Western diet, they become highly susceptible to it.

Homocysteine

In 1969, Dr. Kilmer McCully, a pathologist at Massachusetts General Hospital in Boston, was investigating the death of an eight-year-old boy. The boy had suffered a stroke—quite a rare occurrence in such a young child. Dr. McCully came away with no real answers, but the case came back to haunt him when the boy's sister suffered a heart attack several years later, when she was in her thirties. When he examined the girl, he noticed that the lens of one of her eyes had become dislocated. He recalled having recently read a paper in a Scandinavian medical journal that had discussed a rare genetic disease that caused lens dislocation. The article had said that those born with the disease could be identified by high levels of a protein called "homocysteine" in their urine.

After some more medical detective work, Dr. McCully found that both the boy and his sister did indeed have high levels of homocysteine, along with serious cases of premature atherosclerosis. He developed a theory that some kind of causal link existed between high homocysteine and blood vessel disease. When Dr. McCully presented this idea to his superiors, he was rewarded as innovators often are by the administrators who run major medical centers: He was fired. Nonplussed, he moved to a Veterans' Administration hospital in Rhode Island where he quietly engaged in twenty years of experimentation that would ultimately provide sound support for the homocysteine–heart disease connection. A growing body of research continues to give credence to Dr. McCully's theories.

Homocysteine is one of many amino acids that the body uses to build proteins. It is not found in the diet, but is produced in the body as a key compound for forming the amino acid "methionine," as well as cystathione, which is converted to an important antioxidant called "gluta thione." Cells require these amino acids for the manufacture of glutathione and new genetic material. The conversion of homocysteine into methionine and cystathione is orchestrated by three of the B vitamins: folate, vitamin B_{12}, and vitamin B_6.

Plant proteins, by comparison with meat proteins, contain much less methionine. Since the ancient human diet was plant-based, there was much less methionine than in today's diet, and genes were selected that optimized the ability of the body to make methionine from homocysteine.

The enzymes that performed this function were helped by B vitamins and folic acid, which were also present in large amounts in plant foods. Today, the diet is the opposite of the ancient diet by being rich in methionine and poor in folic acid. About 10 percent of the population have an inherited tendency, based on several different genes, to have higher than normal homocysteine levels. Once again, modern man's diet has resulted in a gene-diet imbalance.

When people who have suffered heart attacks are given an intravenous dose of methionine, between 25 and 40 percent end up with high homocysteine levels. This is a good indication that they are genetically susceptible to high homocysteine when they eat too many methionine-rich foods (meats and dairy products) and not enough B_6 and folic acid–rich foods (vegetables and whole grains). Researchers are moving closer to an understanding of the exact mutations that cause homocysteine levels to rise. Lack of sufficient folate, B_6, and B_{12} in the diet can bring out an individual's tendency toward high homocysteine levels by slowing the conversion of homocysteine to methionine.

Scandinavian women are more likely than others to have a rare immune disease that prevents them from absorbing B_{12} in the gut. This defect causes pernicious anemia, a rare form of B_{12} deficiency. People over the age of sixty-five also may have problems absorbing vitamin B_{12}. There is an important relationship between vitamin B_{12} and folate. Folate will cause nerve damage when it is taken in large amounts (400 to 1,000 micrograms) only in situations where vitamin B_{12} deficiency exists on a genetic or dietary basis. It's easy for your physician to test for vitamin B_{12} deficiency and pernicious anemia during a routine visit, and the problem is just as easily remedied with regular B_{12} injections or with a sublingual (dissolved under the tongue) or intranasal (dropped into the nose) version of the vitamin. Taken in these ways, B_{12} passes directly into the bloodstream without having to be absorbed in the stomach.

Just as the diabetic's genetic tendency to accumulate fat comes back to haunt him in the modern era of food excess, so, too, does the modern-day increase in methionine intake and decrease in folate and B_6 consumption result in an increased risk of heart disease. High homocysteine levels have also been linked to DNA damage and a higher risk of cancer.

Fibrinogen, Inflammation, and Infection

Fibrinogen is a protein found in the blood that is necessary for the formation of clots. Chronically elevated levels of fibrinogen have been shown to increase heart disease risk about twofold. Men tend to have higher fibrinogen levels than women, and African Americans have higher levels than Caucasians.

Smoking raises fibrinogen counts, and quitting causes them to drop. In the famous Framingham study, which examined lifestyle and diet choices in thousands of men in order to find associations between these variables and the risk of heart disease, about half of the increased heart disease risk attributable to smoking could be blamed on elevated fibrinogen. Advancing age, obesity, diabetes, menopause, and high LDL—all of which increase heart disease risk—are associated with increased fibrinogen.

The process of breaking up clots in the blood, called "fibrinolysis," has been shown to be impaired in those at high risk of heart disease. The greatest number of heart attacks occur at nine o'clock on Monday mornings, and it turns out that the platelets—the blood cells that work with fibrinogen to form clots—are stickiest at this particularly stressful time of the week. Exercise, weight loss, and smoking cessation are usually enough to bring fibrinogen levels down and restore normal fibrinolysis.

Blood clotting is also affected by the process of inflammation. Inflammation is the redness, heat, swelling, and pain that occurs in an area of injury, infection, or irritation. White blood cells and fluid collect and cause swelling, which in turn causes pain, heat, and redness. While inflammation can be bothersome, it's necessary; it's one of the ways in which the body heals itself.

Inflammation doesn't always occur where you can see it. At any given time, pockets of inflammation can be found throughout your body, doing maintenance work wherever it's needed. Sometimes, the inflammatory response goes too far, so that a process meant to heal ends up doing harm to healthy tissues. Autoimmune diseases, such as rheumatoid arthritis, lupus, and Crohn's disease, are examples of an overactive and misdirected inflammatory process.

Plaque formation in the coronary arteries is an inflammatory process. Increased levels of C-reactive protein, a marker of inflammation, were found to be associated with a three- to fivefold increase in heart disease risk in two major studies from the Harvard School of Public Health. These studies suggest that the immune system has sensed some injury to the heart's blood vessels that requires repair. White blood cells are drawn to the inner surface of the coronary arteries, where they stick before migrating into the blood vessel wall to take up cholesterol. Specialized proteins in the blood, called "intercellular adhesion molecules," take part in the inflammatory process, increasing the stickiness of the inner surface of blood vessels. Interestingly, these same molecules play a role in cancer formation. High rates of both heart disease and cancer are found in the same countries around the world, and evidence is strong that inflammation and infection contribute to the onset and progression of both diseases.

New research is revealing that chronic infections and heart disease often exist in the same people. Such infections include *Chlamydia pneumoniae*, usually associated with pelvic infections; *Helicobacter pylori*, associated with stomach ulcers and stomach cancer; *Herpesvirus hominis*, the cause of cold sores and genital herpes; and cytomegalovirus, usually transmitted from cat feces to humans. While they may not cause overt signs of infectious disease in those who harbor them, they have all been found trapped in plaques lining the coronary arteries. It may be that they have simply been caught there, but it may also be that they act to stimulate the immune system and set the inflammatory process in motion.

Here, again, we see a clash between genes and environment. Humankind fought infectious diseases in an environment of undernutrition for millennia, and having active inflammatory and clotting systems provided good defenses against infection. The modern diet—unbalanced in fat types compared to our ancient plant-based diet—interacts with these highly sensitive systems in such a way as to push inflammation beyond a healthful balance so that a process meant to protect and heal us can end up causing great harm.

Aspirin is a blood-thinning drug that controls inflammation and is amazingly effective in the prevention of heart disease. Aspirin can also inhibit the growth of colon cancer—another sign that cancer and heart disease share inflammation as a common root cause. Take a baby aspirin or half an adult aspirin a day if it doesn't irritate your stomach. And new COX-2 inhibitor drugs, which also fight inflammation, are being studied as potential therapies for cancer and heart disease.

The Benefits of Plant Foods

There are many different benefits of increasing fruit and vegetable intake to prevent heart disease. First, you reduce the number of calories you are eating overall by displacing high-fat/high-sweet snacks with foods that have fewer calories per bite. Second, you reduce the overload of omega-6 fatty acids and balance them with more omega-3 fatty acids. Third, you obtain the benefits of the many antioxidant chemicals that give these foods their individual bright colors. Fourth, you increase the fiber in your diet, including the soluble fibers that bind cholesterol particles in the intestine and remove them from your body. Fifth, you increase your intake of phytosterol from certain vegetables, and these compounds compete with cholesterol for absorption into your body. So you can see that by eating the nutritional rainbow—the seven families of plant foods you have learned about—you will be reducing your risk of heart disease.

Heart Disease Can Be Prevented

Enormous progress has already been made in the fight against heart disease. In my early days as an interning physician, most of the heart attack patients I saw were forty-five-year-old men who were forty or more pounds overweight and had been eating a high-fat diet and smoking. Today, as consciousness about healthy diet and lifestyle habits rises, first heart attacks are more likely to strike seventy-five and eighty-year-olds.

Clearly, heart disease doesn't commonly occur out of the blue. Genes and nutrients interact in many ways to set the stage for a heart attack. The more we learn about these interactions, the better able we are to work toward prevention.

12

Cancer Is a DNA Disease

J ust as human beings live and die in a cycle of life that maintains the world's population, almost all normal cells in your body live for a certain period of time and then die. This cellular life cycle allows the constant renewal of tissues to take place in your body. New, healthy cells replace old ones, maintaining the function of all of your organ systems.

The life expectancy of every cell is programmed into its genes. Programmed cell death is called "apoptosis," a word you will hear more frequently in the future in relation to cancer. Mutations can change those genes, turning off apoptosis and causing the cell to multiply and grow continually. If normal cells are grown in a test tube, they will divide about twenty times before they die. While many genetic mutations are meaningless or harmless, and many can be repaired, certain kinds of mutations can cause a cell to fail to die on schedule. The mutated cell comprises the very beginnings of a cancerous tumor, which under the right conditions will grow and spread. Cancer cells can reproduce an unlimited number of times. In laboratories all over the world, scientists study the cell lines of cancer patients who have long since died from their disease.

These types of mutations aren't passed from parent to child; they are a response of an individual's inherited genetic makeup to his or her environment. Most cancers originate with genetic mutations in the cells of organs where the cells replace themselves at a rapid clip throughout life: the breasts, the reproductive organs, the colon, the skin, the intestines, the lungs, and the bladder. The chances of carcinogenic mutations are greater in these tissues simply by virtue of the fact that they reproduce their DNA more frequently than other cells do, making mistakes in replication more likely.

Mutations that lead to cancer also originate in parts of the body that are frequently exposed to toxins or high levels of hormones that enhance cell growth: the colon, the prostate, the ovaries, the uterus. Such mutations naturally occur often, but only a small percentage of those mutated cells go on to cause a cancer that will go through the steps of progression, invasion, and metastasis—processes you will learn more about as you read on. As is the case with heart disease, obesity, and diabetes, the genes that happen to increase susceptibility to cancer evolved to serve other purposes: most likely, to deal with the wide variety of phytochemicals found in the ancient hunter-gatherer diet.

Common genetic variations (polymorphisms) from person to person can mean that one won't develop cancer under the same circumstances that will bring out cancerous changes in another. This is why lung cancer doesn't strike every smoker. Specific genetic fingerprints are associated with up to double the risk of cancer, but that risk can be controlled with dietary changes. In rare instances cancer can be traced back to a single faulty gene inherited from the parents, but it is most often complex interactions between diet, genes, and environment that encourage the growth of cancer along every step of the process.

Cancer Is a Disease of Civilization

The average human life span has increased significantly with the improvements in infant mortality, sanitation, and nutrition in developing countries. As infectious disease has become less of a danger, chronic diseases associated with aging have become more common. Cancer is probably the most feared of these diseases.

Every seventeen seconds a baby boomer reaches the age of fifty. Some 76 million Americans are now over the age of fifty. It is estimated that in the next ten years, one in three women and one in two men over fifty will be diagnosed with cancer. Fortunately, the diagnosis of cancer is no longer necessarily a terminal decree because of prevention, early diagnosis, and more effective therapies. In the best-case scenario, early detection of a cancer serves as a much-needed wake-up call to those who could be taking better care of themselves.

Cancer rates are five to fifteen times higher in developed nations than in developing ones. In parts of the world where the diet consists mostly of fresh fruits and vegetables and whole grains—in contrast to the typical Western diet of fatty meats, refined flours, oils, and sugars—the risk of cancer is much lower. When people move from low-risk countries such as Japan to high-risk countries such as the United States, their cancer risk shoots up within a single generation. Obviously, their genes haven't changed that quickly, but the diet they begin to eat upon arriving in the Western world has a potent interaction with their genetic makeup, thus increasing their susceptibility to cancer.

There are many studies that suggest that through changes in diet and lifestyle it is indeed possible to interfere with the development, growth, and spread of cancer even after it has been discovered and treated by using chemotherapy, surgery, or radiation. In the next few decades, the science of oncology (cancer medicine) will continue to develop new approaches to cancer prevention, early diagnosis, and treatment, buying time for cancer patients to make the changes in their diets and lifestyles that will help prevent or delay the fatal spread and progression of cancer in the body.

How Cancer Grows and Spreads

Here's the short course on how cancer goes from a single cell to a systemic disease. Dietary choices and genes contribute differently at each of these stages of cancer development:

1. Initiation/abnormal cell growth: A mutation in one or more normal cells initiates the cancer, and each division of the cell replicates mutated genes and accumulates additional genetic mutations. At this point, either the body's defenses target and eliminate that cell or group of cells, or they reproduce to form a primary tumor.

2. Progression and invasion: The group of abnormal cells continues to divide and spread, forming a primary tumor. The tumor

begins to grow its own blood vessels, invade neighboring tissues, and interfere with organ function.

3. Metastasis: Cells break off the tumor and travel through the blood and lymph systems to organ systems outside the one in which the primary tumor developed. They lodge there, continuing to divide and overtake healthy tissues. Specialized proteins stimulate the growth of new blood vessels to feed these new tumors, and other proteins extend the invasion of the primary tumor and metastases into adjacent tissues. This process has been likened to the initial changes that occur when a fertilized egg implants in the uterus.

As cancer cells grow, they cross boundaries that separate tissues and organs from one another. Specific tumors travel to specific tissues; for example, prostate cancer usually spreads to the bones of the spine, while colon cancer usually spreads to the liver. Once they have grown and spread enough for symptoms to arise, cancerous growths can cause internal bleeding, infection, or organ failure.

Metastasis means that the cancer is spreading aggressively. The human cancer cell lines being grown in laboratories are usually taken from metastases. Metastases grow better outside the body than do cells from the original (primary) tumor. When primary breast tumor cells from humans are implanted in mice, they grow best when implanted in the mammary-fat pads. The cells will take hold and form tumors if implanted in other areas, but they grow differently.

Genetic influences on metastasis are quite complex and not well understood. They include extensive mutations in cancer cells and other cells that confer a growth advantage to the cancer, genes that code for DNA repair, genes that affect the activity of the immune system, and genes that code for the growth of new blood vessels to nourish expanding tumors. It's possible that cancer medicine will find ways to affect these genetic influences, slowing the spread of cancer through the body.

High Risk, Low Risk: The Roles of Diet and Environment

It is a well-known fact that the risk of cancer is greater in some countries than in others. When victims of accidental death from high-risk and low-risk parts of the world are autopsied, the number of microscopic breast or prostate cancers found in their bodies is similar. In other words, the formation of cancerous cells in certain areas of the body is a phenomenon that happens universally, as part of the normal aging process in humans. Autopsies performed on twenty- to thirty-year-olds usually demonstrate that there are no prostate tumors. At between forty and sixty years of age, precancerous lesions are found in accident victims, and above age sixty a significant number of normal men have tiny prostate cancers, found incidentally in autopsies. The number of tumors that grow to clinically detectable dimensions, however, is five to ten times higher in the high-risk nations than in the low-risk nations. When people in low-risk countries do develop cancer, their tumors tend to be less aggressive and slower to spread.

When women migrate from low-risk to high-risk countries, their breast cancer risk increases within fifteen years; the reverse is true with migration from a high-risk to a low-risk country. In humans the process of breast cancer promotion from a single abnormal cell to a detectable tumor is also about fifteen years. It appears that diet has its most significant effects after the cancer has already formed, acting to inhibit or stimulate the growth of that cancer.

The Transformation of a
Pre-Carcinogen into a Carcinogen

It hasn't been easy for scientists to identify which substances are carcinogenic and which are not. This is because many carcinogens only become carcinogenic once they are acted on by the body's detoxification systems (which, you may recall, developed for the purpose of neutralizing toxic chemicals in plant foods). Such substances include pesticides, chemicals from tobacco smoke, chemicals used to smoke and pickle foods, and heterocyclic amines (chemicals that form in cooked meats). These chemicals are acted on by enzymes that transform them into potent carcinogens with strong potential for damaging DNA. While the inheritance of certain forms of these enzymes increases individual susceptibility to developing cancer on exposure to carcinogens, it is possible to reduce exposure either by avoiding these substances altogether or eating foods such as broccoli and Brussels sprouts, which increase the activity of beneficial carcinogen-inactivating enzymes.

Slowing Cancer Growth
with Calorie Restriction

Primary tumor cells depend on interactions with the normal cells around them to maintain their abnormal growth. One of the ways in which nutrition affects cancer growth is by affecting these interactions. We don't know exactly how, and so it's difficult to make specific nutritional recommendations for countering the growth of cancer once it has become advanced. One tactic that has worked in animal studies to slow cancer growth at every stage is calorie restriction.

Over two hundred breast cancer studies have been carried out using a carcinogenic chemical called DMBA. When DMBA is instilled into the stomachs of female rats at fifty-five days of age, it links to DNA on chromosome twelve and leads to breast cancer in every single animal given the DMBA. If DMBA is given before the forty-eighth day or after the sixty-second day of age, it doesn't cause breast cancer in the rats. Sexual maturation occurs at about twenty-one days of age in female rats, but their breasts don't mature until around fifty-five days. During this time there is a burst of cell replication in the breast tissue as the milk ducts form.

While all of the animals exposed to DMBA at the appropriate time will ultimately develop breast cancer, there are nutritional strategies that can delay its onset. In rats put on a low-calorie diet, far fewer tumors have formed at twenty weeks after the DMBA is administered. The degree to which tumor formation is inhibited depends on the degree of calorie restriction. Significant decreases in cancer growth are seen with as little as a 12 percent reduction in calorie intake, while a 40 percent calorie restriction leads to about a 60 percent inhibition of tumor growth compared with animals allowed to eat as much as they liked. It is important to note that these dietary changes delayed the onset of detectable tumor growth in a situation where the mutation that causes cancer has been created in 100 percent of the animals. In humans such a delay could theoretically permit a cancer patient to survive long enough to die of something else.

Oxidation, Antioxidants, and Cancer

As cells grow they "turn on" processes that produce free radicals, the highly reactive oxygen atoms carrying an extra electron that were discussed earlier. Free radicals can do serious damage to structures within cells, including DNA. They can also induce gene mutations that lead to cancer.

Cells have defense mechanisms against free radicals. When they are exposed to a pro-oxidant—a substance that accelerates free-radical formation—their genes respond in six places on two different chromosomes. These genes trigger the production within the cells of the chemicals called "antioxidants." Antioxidants can act to neutralize free radicals before they do any real damage.

While many antioxidants can be made in the body, others must be absorbed from the foods we eat; still others are both made in the body *and* obtained from the diet. Most of the antioxidants we eat come from fruits and vegetables. By studying the free-radical-neutralizing effects of various antioxidants in laboratory experiments, we can tell which are best at keeping oxidation under control.

Plants evolved in an atmosphere that contained no oxygen. As they converted sunlight into energy, absorbing carbon dioxide and producing oxygen, the increasing concentration of oxygen in the atmosphere poisoned their cells. Antioxidant defenses in plants were developed in response to this atmospheric shift. When we eat plant foods, we benefit from these chemicals that originally evolved to benefit the plant itself.

Experiments on animals have shown us that a deficiency of antioxidants can lead to cancer, and that giving the animals supplemental antioxidants can inhibit the process of cancer development. When tumors are removed from animals depleted of antioxidants (or depleted of nutrients needed to make antioxidants in their own cells), examination shows that their cells have been subjected to very active oxidation and DNA damage. Giving these animals extra vitamin C or vitamin E can inhibit the process of cancer growth. The DNA-damaging and carcinogenic effects of suboptimal amounts of dietary antioxidants are likely to promote cancer development in humans and in laboratory mice.

Why Tobacco Doesn't Always Cause Cancer

Both animal experiments and studies of genetics in populations lend support to the idea that certain people are predisposed to cancer by overly active liver detoxification systems. Active liver detoxification systems were perfectly suited to dealing with the large quantity of plant chemicals, both harmful and helpful, found in the ancient diet. In modern times a lack of fruits and vegetables leaves these enzymes with nothing to do but activate carcinogens by oxidizing polyunsaturated fats, chemicals from charred meats, and other dietary and environmental toxins. Excessive activation can transform otherwise harmless chemicals into potent carcinogens.

When scientists began to study the connection between tobacco smoke and lung cancer, they had to take into account the fact that some people who smoke don't ever get the disease. Smoking accounts for 85 percent of all lung cancer and about 35 percent of all cancers, but not every smoker ends up with lung cancer. There are probably many genes that increase susceptibility to lung cancer among smokers. We are a long way from identifying them all, but a few are becoming well understood.

A protein called an "aryl hydrocarbon receptor (AhR)," which sits on the surface of lung cells, appears to be involved in the lung cancer–smoking relationship. About 15 percent of normal individuals have genes that code for a form of AhR with a higher affinity for the cancer-causing chemicals in smoke. This means that they are more likely to bind AhR in vulnerable cells, creating adducts that significantly increase the risk of lung cancer among smokers.

When I began to examine this research, it occurred to me that the aryl hydrocarbon receptor could not possibly have evolved to bind the chemicals in tobacco smoke, since there was no tobacco fifty thousand years ago. This receptor must have evolved to bind to a particular chemical found in plant foods. This receptor actually binds a variety of substances in addition to the chemicals found in cigarette smoke. When our laboratory caused liver cancers by restricting the intake of methionine, folic acid, and choline, the liver cells had excessive amounts of the aryl hydrocarbon receptor and the enzyme called "cytochrome P450 1A1," which activates the chemicals in cigarette smoke to form potent carcinogens.

Dietary Patterns That Increase Cancer Risk

In the future we will be able to measure changes in the genes that occur before cancer ever develops—a type of early detection that will greatly improve modern medicine's ability to prevent this disease. We will be able to identify people who have gene polymorphisms that mean greater cancer risk, such as variations in the genes that code for enzymes that activate carcinogens or fail to repair DNA. Those individuals may be at higher risk of developing cancer than others, even when they are all eating the same foods and are all exposed to the same environmental toxins.

This doesn't mean our hands are tied until those discoveries are made. It is estimated that one third of all cases of cancer are attributable to dietary factors. Nutrition is especially strongly implicated in cancers of the stomach, colon, breast, and prostate. There are common dietary patterns that increase cancer risk in most people, and enough is known about those patterns to merit making some changes now. Overnutrition (eating too many calories), lack of antioxidant nutrients from fruits and vegetables, and fatty-acid imbalances can stimulate cells to replicate more frequently, increasing the chances that a critical mutation will convert a normal cell into a cancerous one.

Obesity. The American Cancer Society sponsored a study almost thirty years ago to find out what lifestyle habits might increase cancer risk. This enormous research effort, involving 750,000 people, found that obesity significantly increased the risk of breast, colon, ovarian, uterine, pancreatic, kidney, and gallbladder cancer.

Lack of fruits and vegetables. Studies of populations around the world— particularly those that take into account what happens when members of one population migrate to another area—have provided a great deal of evidence that people who consume about a pound of fruits and vegetables daily have markedly lower risks of lung, esophageal, and stomach cancers. Even smokers benefit from the phytochemicals in fruits and vegetables: Japanese who eat green and yellow vegetables and smoke have less lung cancer than those who smoke and don't eat these foods.

All in all, over seventy studies strongly implicate fruits and vegetables as important cancer preventives. Twenty-eight of thirty studies on stomach cancer, fifteen of nineteen studies on colon cancer, twelve of fourteen studies on esophageal cancer, eleven of thirteen studies on lung cancer, and nine of thirteen studies on breast cancer show that if you eat your vegetables and fruits every day, your chances of avoiding cancer are much improved.

Lack of micronutrients. At each step of the process of cancer development, growth, and spread, diet clearly has multiple influences. In the spirit of the "magic bullet" philosophy embraced by modern, pharmaceutically biased medicine, researchers have been examining specific micronutrient components of nutritious foods to discover exactly which chemicals are responsible for the beneficial effects. Micronutrients include vitamins, minerals, and phytochemicals (chemicals found in plants that aren't vitamins or minerals, but which have distinct effects in the body).

Plant foods, including fruits, vegetables, spices, herbs, and whole grains, are the best food sources of cancer-preventive micronutrients. Fruits and vegetables contain phytochemicals and other bioactive compounds shown to have anti-inflammatory, antioxidant, and anti-tumor effects.

Cancer-Preventive Effects of Some Micronutrients

Micronutrient	*Effect*
Calcium *(supplement)*	Inhibits the uptake of carcinogen from the intestines; slows the rate of division of normal cells in the gut to prevent development of colon polyps and cancer.
Tea polyphenols (green and black teas) *(supplement)*	Act as very potent antioxidants and inhibit the growth of new-tumor blood vessels. Oppose cancer-promoting hormone actions in some cases.
Sulforaphane *(green)*	Enhances the breakdown and excretion of carcinogens in the liver.
Ellagic acid *(red/purple)*	Prevents the binding of carcinogens to DNA.
Limonoids *(yellow/orange)*	Inhibits cholesterol synthesis needed to activate cancer cell growth
Vitamin E *(whole grains, nuts, seeds)*	Neutralizes free radicals involved in the process of tumor growth and development; strengthens the immune system (which plays an important role in the fight against cancer).

Micronutrient	Effect
Carotenoids *(orange; red; yellow/green)*	Improve communication between cells, which helps them fight the spread of cancer.
Genistein (one of the *soy isoflavones*) *(protein)*	Induces programmed cell death, reminding cells that they need to die to make way for new, healthier cells; inhibits the growth of new blood vessels that form to feed a growing tumor.
Garlic allyl sulfides *(white/green)*	Modify activity of DNA polymerase.
Folic acid *(yellow/green)*	Corrects imbalances in DNA methylation.

These compounds, which comprise a virtual anticancer pharmacy, affect the process of cancer formation and growth in far more ways than we have yet discovered. Some of these nutrients are now available in the form of supplements, but none of these acts as a "magic bullet" by itself to ensure lifelong freedom from cancer. When considering the ideal cancer-preventive diet, it makes sense to look at the whole diet—a combination of many different foods containing many different compounds—rather than trying to isolate single nutrients as preventives or cures.

Some micronutrients inhibit tumor initiation by preventing carcinogenic chemicals from coming into contact with DNA. This can be accomplished by blocking the activation of a chemical that becomes carcinogenic only when activated (often referred to as a "pro-carcinogen"). Isothiocyanate, a phytochemical found in broccoli, does just this by inhibiting the action of cytochrome P450 on pro-carcinogens. A large family of chemical compounds called "glucosinolates," found in 450 different plant species, can be converted into isothiocyanates in the body. The estimated daily intake of glucosinolates is about 30 milligrams in the United States and Canada and about 112 milligrams in Japan.

Blocking agents can also work by increasing the rate at which cancer-causing chemicals are broken down, or by trapping those chemicals so that they can't go to work creating cancer cells. Phytochemicals in green onions, red cabbage, kale, Brussels sprouts, and broccoli significantly speed up the action of enzymes that break down carcinogens.

Many of the plant chemicals being studied today have more than one anticancer effect. Sulforaphane, a phytochemical in Brussels sprouts and broccoli that induces higher enzyme activity, also works as an antioxidant while stimulating the formation of another antioxidant, glutathione.

Cancer researchers often ask me why we shouldn't simply isolate the active agent from a food in order to make a new drug. My answer to them is that the interactions of nutrients with each other are critical to their effects on the precancerous or cancerous cell. The process of carcinogenesis is a complicated one that incorporates many steps, and whole food works in multiple ways, modifying elements of each step of that process.

I often use the example of cancer chemotherapy, where the use of several drugs—each of which works by a different mechanism—is often much more potent than a single drug. Multidrug chemotherapy is usually the best choice for cancer treatment when aggressive therapy is needed. This was discovered after oncologists experimented with a combination of drugs to treat Hodgkin's lymphoma. Since this regimen, known as MOPP (an acronym for the names of the drugs used), was developed, similar approaches have been used for most common cancers.

Scientists don't care for solutions like this because they are used to doing research in a specific way: They compare the effects of a single drug or nutrient with the effects of no treatment at all. A change in research methods will be required in order to study the effects of whole foods on cancer risk and cancer progression. My belief is that the use of biomarkers, physiological measurements that show us how well a treatment works, will be an important part of these research methods. Just as cholesterol is a useful biomarker for determining how diet affects the risk for heart disease, I believe biomarkers for cancer risk and disease progression will be developed. Today, markers such as PSA (prostate specific antigen) are useful in following the clinical course of prostate cancer, but have not been shown to be affected by diet.

Fats and Fatty-Acid Balance

A considerable number of studies have shown links between total fat intake and cancer. Homer Black, M.D., at Baylor College of Medicine, and colleagues conducted a study of skin cancer patients where half ate a high-fat diet and half shifted to a low-fat diet, and found that the number of new skin cancers in the low-fat group was a fraction of the number that developed in the high-fat group. Fats can work to enhance the formation and spread of cancer in many ways: Unsaturated fats from vegetable and seed oils can become oxidized, introducing an overload of free radicals into the body. Eating a diet high in fats can contribute to over-nutrition and obesity, because fats contain more than twice as many calories per gram as proteins or carbohydrates.

Recent advances in cancer research have revealed that it may not only be the total amount of fat but the *type* of fat that makes the difference. Changing the type of dietary fat in lab animals' feed has distinct effects on tumor growth. More dietary oils rich in omega-6 fatty acids promote tumor growth, while oils providing more omega-3 fatty acids inhibit tumor growth. In animals with poor immune function, implanted human tumors spread when they are fed omega-6-rich feed, but not when they are fed feed rich in omega-3s. This makes good physiologic sense, considering that omega-3s have anti-inflammatory effects that oppose the pro-inflammatory effects of omega-6 fats. The link between cancer and inflammation has garnered considerable interest in scientific circles since the publication of studies on the cancer-inhibiting effects of aspirin and other nonsteroidal anti-inflammatory drugs (NSAIDs). Prednisone, a powerful anti-inflammatory steroid drug, is sometimes prescribed by oncologists to slow cancer growth.

Modulating Immune Function
with Pro-biotic Bacteria

Bacteria far outnumber any other organism on the face of the earth. Each human being is playing host to about 100 billion bacteria. These highly adaptive microscopic organisms live in perfect harmony with us and the other animals around us.

Most are benign, and some are actually a natural and helpful part of human physiology. Bacteria work for us in two ways: Some strains stimulate the immune system of growing children to develop strong defenses, while other strains take up residence in the gastrointestinal tract, forming a symbiotic relationship with their human hosts. They help digest certain fibers and other foods we cannot eat, and these chemicals produced by bacteria can promote normal cell growth in the colon.

Modern technology has made it possible to create a germ-free environment. When animals are raised in this sort of environment, they don't develop healthy immune systems, but easily develop infections as soon as they are removed from it. Animals raised under normal conditions, in the presence of bacteria, develop stronger immune systems that can defend them against all manner of bacterial threats. Exposure to bacteria "trains" the young immune system.

In the era before refrigeration, so-called healthy bacteria were cultivated in milk in order to preserve it. Cottage cheese, yogurt, and buttermilk were the products of this fermentation process. When these foods are eaten, several strains of these bacteria—including *Lactobacillus acidophilus* and *Lactobacillus bifidus*—colonize the gut. There they stimulate immune function and compete with any unhealthy bacteria or other organisms that try to invade the intestines.

While we aren't sure what role these unhealthy bacteria and other organisms play in causing and promoting cancer, research has shown that people who eat pro-biotic-containing foods regularly live longer and may be at decreased risk of certain cancers. In 1908 a Russian scientist ascribed the longevity enjoyed by Bulgarian peasants to their habit of eating yogurt and other fermented dairy products.

A more direct cancer-preventive effect of pro-biotics is their ability to prevent the formation of carcinogens in the colon. When bile acids, which play a role in digestion, pass into the colon, unhealthy colon bacteria can transform them into carcinogenic secondary bile acids. Pro-biotics naturally oppose this process. They also produce short-chain fatty acids such as butyric acid, which act to regulate normal colon cell growth and death; and they absorb and metabolize potentially carcinogenic chemicals. Carcinogens formed in the colon can directly damage the DNA of colon cells, thus promoting colon cancer. Fermentation of milk also predigests the milk sugars (lactose) it contains. This is why many lactose-intolerant people can eat live-culture yogurt without any problem. Live-culture yogurt, some cottage cheeses, kefir, and sweet acidophilus milk are excellent sources of pro-biotics.

The Importance of Early Detection

With modern medical technology, we are able to identify and treat cancers earlier than ever before. We have mammography for breast cancer detection, PSA levels for prostate cancer detection, Pap smears for cervical cancer detection, colonoscopy for colon cancer detection, and endometrial biopsy for the detection of uterine cancer. Tumors can be caught quite early in their development with these tests. When coupled with preventive measures—eating right for your genes—early detection and treatment can mean a complete cure.

13

Aging, Sex Drive, Mental Function, and Your DNA

Life has been cynically characterized as a sexually transmitted disease that is uniformly fatal. However, modern medical advances may someday make it possible for us to slow the aging process itself, as if it were actually a chronic disease. The goal of aging research is to help humans live as long as possible, with the best quality of life, so that death occurs only after a maximum life span has been enjoyed.

Why Do We Age?

Why do we age? This question has intrigued humankind since the beginnings of recorded history. Why hasn't nature's design allowed us to live out our life spans in good health, with skin taut, eyes bright, joints flexible, mind sharp, hair its original color, muscles firm, energy high? What exactly goes on in the aging body at the cellular level, and is there any way to slow it down or stop it in its tracks? We are a long way from any definitive answers, but experiments in laboratories around the world on worms, fruit flies, and mice are helping us to understand some of the basic processes that cause aging.

Anyone over forty can attest to the fact that aging changes your body and mind in a great many ways, some subtle, some not so subtle. Most of us know people who look and behave as though they were much younger than their biological age, and others who we might guess to be far older than they really are. Genetic variation accounts for some of these differences, but gene-nutrient interaction has significant effects as well. This is particularly true of certain age-related diseases: osteoporosis, various forms of mental deterioration or dementia (including Alzheimer's disease), and the age-related eye diseases, cataracts and macular degeneration.

We Are Living Longer Than Ever

Despite our ignorance as to the whys and wherefores of the aging process, humans have enjoyed significant increases in life span since our earliest days on earth. Your chances of living beyond your mid-twenties during the Roman Empire were slim. If you were born around the end of the nineteenth century, you could expect to survive into your mid-forties. Those born in the early twentieth century had an average life span of sixty to seventy years, and a child born today could very well live to be over a hundred. Increases in the human life span up until the twentieth century have been mostly attributable to improvements in the prevention and treatment of infectious diseases and premature heart disease.

The maximum recorded human life span is 122 years and 6 months. There have been reports that haven't been proved because of lack of birth records of people living nearly 130 years. As we move toward a deeper understanding of the aging process, the average life span will lengthen, and perhaps one day it will come close to what we now consider the absolute maximum number of years a human being can live—in good health and in sound mind.

Theories of Aging

Aging is much more than simple wear and tear on the body. You may have heard the story about the elderly woman who goes to her doctor with a sore right knee. After examining her the doctor gently tells her that there isn't much to be done, that these aches and pains are just a part of growing old. She answers, "So you say, but my left knee is just as old as my right one, and it feels just fine!"

Scientists have investigated a number of leads in their quest to unlock the secrets of why we age. They have arrived at a few promising conclusions, all of which make good physiological sense but which leave unanswered questions. In all probability each of these theories has some truth to it, and further discoveries will show us how they fit together.

Telomere Shortening

With each normal division of a cell, a small piece of genetic material at one end of the DNA strand is lost. These bits of DNA at the ends of chromosomes are called "telomeres." The loss of a small amount of the telomere with each cell division programs normal cells so that after twenty divisions they can no longer divide. At this point normal cells die to make way for younger cells. Telomerase is an enzyme that adds DNA back onto the strand following each cell division. The genetic equipment needed to make telomerase is found in nearly every cell, but something renders it inactive in all cells other than cancer cells, sperm cells, and the cells that regenerate the intestinal lining. Telomerase activity allows cells to reproduce indefinitely—to cheat death.

You may have noticed certain trends toward longevity, or the lack thereof, in your family. If your grandparents and their siblings lived into their eighties or nineties, your chances of doing so are greater than if they died young. Wouldn't it be interesting, asked some gene researchers, if we could estimate longevity based on the length of a person's telomeres? It seemed a sensible theory; longer telomeres would mean longer-lived cells, and longer-lived cells would, hypothetically, mean longer life for the organism. When studies were carried out on mice, however, the theory didn't hold up: Strains of mice with long telomeres didn't live any longer than those with average-length telomeres.

There are other holes in the argument that our telomeres decide our life span. While the regulation of telomerase may play some role in aging, the changes we associate with the "golden years"—muscle weakness, arthritis, heart disease, skin and hair changes, and declines in mental function—have been found to be unrelated to telomere shortening. Cancer is characterized by a *lack* of telomere shortening, and it occurs more frequently with aging. There is current research looking into inactivating telomerase as a way of fighting cancer cell growth, but we are a long way from understanding how this process affects human aging.

Cellular Checkpoints and DNA Mutations

Several different theories of aging propose that a key process in aging is damage to mitochondrial and chromosomal DNA. Mitochondria are tiny energy factories in the cells. They have their own DNA, inherited from the mother. Mutations of either chromosomal or mitchochondrial DNA can interfere with the function of the cell. The engine of an old automobile is more likely than a new automobile to create more pollutants when it's running, and with advancing years our mitochondrial engines shift in the same way. As we age our mitochondria become less efficient, producing more free radicals in their day-to-day work of transforming sugars into energy. It is likely that a number of changes in our genes accumulate as we age as a result of the release of excess oxidant molecules from the mitochondria combined with a reduced ability to neutralize these chemicals.

A recent study at the Scripps Research Institute in La Jolla, California, examined the effects of aging on six thousand different genes called "fibroblasts" in skin cells taken from young, middle-aged, and elderly humans, and from children with a rare genetic disease called "progeria." Progeria is a tragic disease in children of premature aging, with graying and thinning of the hair, wrinkling of the skin, arthritis, heart disease, and early death. The scientists found that cells from children with progeria had many of the same genetic mutations as cells from very elderly individuals, while none of these changes were found in young, healthy, normal individuals. With aging there is a silencing of the genes that stimulate DNA repair. Presumably, as a result of the loss of the DNA repair capacity and increased oxidant stress, sixty-one different genes were found to be affected, with over half related to either cell growth and division or the maintenance of the substances surrounding the cell. In this experiment a number of the genes observed to be affected by aging are known to be important for quality control within the cell. They are called "checkpoint genes" since they make the decision, after a cell divides, as to whether it is still functioning well enough to survive. Checkpoint genes weed out the cells most apt to malfunction, and if their activity slows down, quality control suffers.

Calorie Restriction Retards Aging

Overnutrition plays a significant role in premature aging. The more you eat, the more free radicals your mitochondria will produce as you metabolize the calories. Restricting calories reduces metabolic rate and slows the production of free radicals. When Dr. Roy Walford at UCLA restricted the calorie intake of mice by 40 percent and supplemented their diet with vitamins and minerals, they lived twice as long, had better immune function, and had fewer cancers than mice allowed to eat as much as they liked; this was probably due to the decreased free-radical stress on their bodies. Mice go into puberty later when their calories are restricted, and when fed freely in their cages always become obese in their old age. It is interesting to speculate whether it is calorie restriction, the delay of puberty, or the prevention of obesity that extended lifespan. In humans, there is some evidence that being about 10 percent below average weight is associated with an extended life span. However, life-long malnutrition leading to short stature is not likely to catch on as a popular approach to a longer life.

Antioxidants Slow Aging

Supplemental antioxidants slow the aging of laboratory mice. Dr. Bruce Ames, conducting research at the University of California at Berkeley, gave supplemental alpha lipoic acid and N-acetylcarnitine to aging mice. Alpha lipoic acid and N-acetylcarnitine both act in the shuttling of sugars and fats into the mitochondria, where they are broken down for energy. Dr. Ames then examined their liver cells to see how well their mitochondria were functioning, and found that they operated more efficiently, producing fewer free radicals.

Alpha lipoic acid also acts within the antioxidant network to increase the amount of cysteine, a sulfur-containing amino acid. The cells need cysteine to make the antioxidant glutathione. Glutathione can restore the function of the antioxidants vitamin E and vitamin C. Once an antioxidant has quenched a free radical, it becomes oxidized itself and needs to be restored to its former state by another antioxidant. This is one reason why it's important to get a good balance of these nutrients from foods, rather than taking large amounts of any one antioxidant in supplement form. Alpha lipoic acid is the exception to this rule—it never needs the help of other antioxidants to continue its work of protecting cells against oxidative damage. Because it is only found in minute amounts in foods, taking supplemental alpha lipoic acid makes sense.

Ideally, we could get all the nutrients we need to counter free-radical stress from a varied diet rich in plant foods. Because we have moved so far from the Garden of Eden and into the stressful, frantically paced, "more is better" lifestyles typical in Westernized nations, and because we are exposed to so many more substances promoting oxidation than our ancestors were, it makes good sense to supplement some of these nutrients.

Extra Muscle, Not Fat, May Be an Advantage

While being overweight is often a liability in the young and the middle-aged, a few extra pounds, at first glance, appear to give the elderly a survival advantage over their very thin and very heavy counterparts. A number of studies seem to show that an increase in the body mass index, or weight for height, improve survival in the elderly. Some geriatrics researchers have interpreted the advantages of increased weight as being due to increased fat and have theorized that fat might cushion a fall that might otherwise cause a hip fracture. However, older individuals who carry a bit of extra weight generally have more muscle and stronger bones. Since you have to fall over to fracture your hip, it may simply be that increased muscle mass provides better balancing ability. Muscle also stores protein reserves, which help to stave off illness and malnutrition—the major health threats of very old age. An elderly person with pneumonia is more likely to survive if he or she has adequate stores of muscle protein, since depletion of muscle protein to 50 percent of normal levels is incompatible with life.

It isn't easy for the elderly to maintain muscle and fat stores. How many overweight or muscular septegenarians or octogenarians have you encountered? Many elderly people lose their appetites and the ability to digest their food efficiently. Decreased blood flow to the intestines slows the undulating movements of the intestinal wall, which leads to slower digestion and the overgrowth of unfriendly bacteria. This is why constipation and indigestion grow worse with age.

Calcium, Vitamin D, and
Vitamin B12 Supplements

With advancing years less stomach acid and intrinsic factor are produced—changes that mean a decrease in calcium, vitamin D, and vitamin B12 absorption. Difficulty with chewing, dry mouth, and changes in the taste buds contribute to the problem of getting adequate nourishment in old age.

Vitamin and mineral supplements, in forms easily absorbed in the digestive tracts of older people, are an important addition to the diet once these changes have taken place. While I am a strong proponent of impeccable dietary habits throughout life, I'm also a realist who sees that supplements are necessary for the elderly, who are unlikely to get what they need without them. Women over fifty need 1,500 milligrams of calcium because the loss of estrogen reduces the efficiency of calcium absorption. Men and women need vitamin D, due to multiple defects with aging in vitamin D formation, absorption, and conversion into active forms. Mild to moderate vitamin D deficiency is not uncommon in elderly women, particularly in geographic areas where winters are long, cold, and overcast. Getting outside in the sun for twenty minutes a day will support vitamin D production, and supplemental vitamin D as well is a good idea for older people.

Living Longer and Feeling Better

Curiously, my obese patients often come from families with tremendous longevity. The ability to starve, build muscle, and resist infections were all an advantage in ancient times. Judging from the long life spans of their less obese, more active ancestors, the genes that predispose these people to weight gain may work in their favor if they can avoid midlife obesity-related diseases. So there may be a rationale for the presence of these genes. When their obesity is left untreated, these patients end up with the usual complaints of high blood pressure, stroke, heart attack, diabetes, premature aging, and premature death.

When you look at those people currently living to be over 100, the main commonality is an independent spirit and great genetics. They tend to eat all kinds of different diets. The ability to extend the average maximum life span, beyond what has already been achieved by counteracting infectious diseases with improved sanitation and nutrition, will require restructuring our diets and lifestyle.

While heart disease, diabetes, and cancer remain at the top of the list of diseases that kill aging people, other age-related diseases can severely affect an older person's enjoyment of life. Blindness, fragile bones, reduced libido, and deteriorating mental function can certainly make the golden years less than golden.

Maintaining Your Vision

Ultraviolet light threatens our vision, and there are several things you can do to maintain your vision as you age. First, get an eye exam from an ophthalmologist to check out your lens, retina, and eye pressure. Second, wear sunglasses whenever you go out in the sun. Third, eat plenty of the *yellow/green* group in the Color Code. While there are genetics involved in cataracts and age-related macular degeneration, AMD, described below, the above are the things you can do to maintain your vision as you age.

Ultraviolet light is the culprit in both cataracts and AMD. Cataracts occur when the clear lenses that lie behind the pupil become fogged and opaque. Excessive exposure to ultraviolet light contributes to cataract formation. AMD causes about 13 million cases of blindness per year in the United States. AMD affects the retina, which lies along the inside of the eyeball, behind the pupil. When light shines through the pupil onto the retina, a series of complex chemical reactions sends electrical impulses to the brain, and the brain translates those impulses into the picture of what you see. The macula is a small area on the retina where the light is concentrated by the lens. Two potent antioxidants, lutein and zeaxanthin, are concentrated in the macula tissue, where they can protect the retina from damage by free radicals. However, if they are not present in adequate amounts, the risk of AMD and deterioration of this area is increased. The result is blurring and eventual loss of central vision, so that a black spot covers the center of the visual field. While it doesn't cause complete blindness—some peripheral vision is retained—advanced AMD makes reading, driving, and other day-to-day tasks impossible.

Taking supplemental lutein can raise lutein levels in the retina, and numerous studies suggest a strong relationship between a high intake of lutein- and zeaxanthin-containing foods and a resistance to AMD. Lutein and zeaxanthin are found in green and yellow vegetables and in nutritional supplements made from the petals of marigold flowers.

Prevent Thinning Bones and Fractures

Osteoporosis was once considered a normal part of aging, with general acceptance of the stooped, shortened stature suffered by the elderly. Today, osteoporosis is a major public-health problem, one that lies at the root of much unnecessary suffering and debility in otherwise healthy older adults. There are more than 25 million older Americans at risk for osteoporosis, and each year more than 12 billion health care dollars go toward the costs of treating osteoporosis-related fractures.

Bone is not inert or static. It is constantly being remodeled, especially in the hips, spine, and extremities. New bone cells replace old ones, and the turnover of these cells allows bones to grow stronger and denser in response to everyday stresses. This is why weight-bearing exercise has the effect of increasing bone density, and why an area of fractured bone is stronger after it repairs itself than it was before the break occurred.

Two types of cells, osteoclasts and osteoblasts, do the work of maintaining bone strength. The osteoclasts break down and digest old bone cells, while the osteoblasts build new ones, a process known as bone turnover. Physical activity, nutrition, and hormone balance decide the balance of osteoclast and osteoblast activity. When the bones, on a regular basis, have to bear the weight of the body during exercise, the bones respond by adding more cells and removing fewer. Inactivity has the opposite effect. When calcium nutrition is inadequate, bone cells are broken down faster than they are built.

Some Plant Estrogens May Help

Over fifty years ago Dr. Fuller Albright, a pioneer researcher in the field of metabolic bone disease, noted that postmenopausal women were losing excessive amounts of calcium in their urine. He suggested that estrogen somehow affected bone metabolism. Today, much scientific support exists for his theory, as we now know that estrogen helps slow bone resorption, the process by which bone cells are broken down. Soy isoflavones are often called "phytoestrogens," but they are not really estrogens. In fact, they act as antiestrogens in the breast and uterus by displacing estrogen from its binding protein, called the alpha estrogen receptor. This antiestrogen effect is often credited as one of the most important properties of soy in accounting for the lower incidence of breast and uterine cancer seen in countries such as Japan, where soy is eaten as a regular part of the diet. There is another receptor, called the beta estrogen receptor, where soy isoflavones have the same effects as estrogen on building bone and counteracting hot flashes that often occur with menopause. Scientists call these actions "selective estrogen response modifiers," or SERMS, and some soy researchers have applied this same terminology to soy protein isoflavones. A chemical formed from plant estrogens called "ipriflavone" is sold as a dietary supplement and has been studied extensively in Europe, where it has been shown to reduce thinning of the bones.

You Have to Fall Over to Break Your Hip

While healthy nutrition is important, maintaining your muscles, especially the big muscles in your legs, is important. It will help to maintain your stability and keep you from falling over—a necessary prerequisite to the most devastating of the osteoporosis-related fractures, the hip fracture. At this point I should also mention not being overmedicated. Antihypertensive drugs and diuretics, drugs that cause water loss, can cause light-headedness. It is important that, with the advice of your physician, you adjust your medication carefully and monitor your blood pressure at home. To prevent falling get up slowly; men should urinate sitting down as they age, especially in the middle of the night when they are most susceptible to falling.

Keep Your Sex Drive

Sex drive in humans is largely psychological. We evolved as one of the few species that has sex for pleasure as well as reproduction. In most species of animals, sexual activity occurs only during ovulation, when fertilization is likely to occur and there is a high probability of success. The sex act itself is abbreviated in most species, since it leaves the mating animals vulnerable to attack by a predator. In humans and a few other species, sexual activity binds couples together to enhance the family structure needed to teach children, during their long period of pre-pubertal life, the many skills needed for survival. Cultural evolution, which sets man apart from other species, occurs as information is passed, in the prepubertal period of life, from one generation to another.

In women ovulation is not predictable and can occur at variable times each month. Sperm can survive in the female abdomen for up to seventy-two hours and still fertilize an egg moving down the fallopian tubes. In hunter-gatherer societies, menopause in women permits the fertile females to return to the fields to gather food, while the young are cared for by a menopausal grandmother or adoptive aunt. This transition in caretaking usually occurs when breast-feeding ends, after about one year. The practice of breast-feeding serves as a natural form of birth control due to cultural taboos against men having sexual intercourse with women who are breast-feeding. This break in reproductive activity essentially spaces children out to every two years, which is good for hunter-gatherers on the move, since children are ambulatory by two years of age.

What is left of reproductive function as you age? In women libido results from testosterone, the male hormone, which is made by the ovary together with estrogen. At menopause the levels of both hormones fall, but in many women the ratio of testosterone to estrogen increases, so sex drive remains strong. In some women a loss of testosterone leads to decreased libido, and these women benefit from testosterone hormone treatments. A testosterone patch, placed on the skin, will, several hours later, increase sex drive in women. Being vital and exercising so that you feel good about your body is also important in being psychologically prepared for continued sexual activity.

Men are less complex. They have continued sex drive as long as they are healthy. Groucho Marx fathered children in his eighties. However, some men develop problems with performance, now referred to as "erec-tile dysfunction" in television commercials. This term has replaced the more scientific term of "impotence." In many men diabetes or atheroscle-rosis can reduce the blood flow to the penis so that spontaneous erections are reduced or absent. Any drug that constricts the valves, trapping blood in the penis, will work to enhance erections. Papaverine injections, Viagra, and mechanical devices all work to increase erections. Libido in men is also psychological, and unrelated to the ability to perform sexu-ally. Being fit and healthy will increase and maintain your sex drive.

What about aphrodisiacs? Most of the stories about aphrodisiacs are just that, stories. The famous "Spanish fly" is made from insects' bodies and is an irritant toxin that has its effects by irritating the urinary tract. It should be avoided, as it can be toxic in large doses. Other stimulants such as chili peppers and chocolate were also hailed as aphrodisiacs but probably had their effect simply as stimulants of the nervous system. Other foods such as avocados, due to their resemblance to sex organs (which were called "testicle fruits" in Spanish), were thought to be aphrodisiacs. But the best diet for maintaining sex drive is the healthy diet you will achieve by using the Color Code.

Maintain Your Memory

With aging, some memory loss is normal. By the fifth or sixth decade of life, the average person has lost up to 20 percent of the neurons in the brain's memory center. However, this inability to remember details is much different from the severe group of diseases called "dementias," which are marked by a general decline in all areas of mental ability. Dementia affects 6 to 10 percent of people aged sixty-five and older. If milder cases of dementia are counted, these prevalence rates double. Alzheimer's disease accounts for two thirds of these cases of demetia.

Alzheimer's Disease and Antioxidants

The brain of a person with Alzheimer's disease looks quite different from the brain of a person without it. When a brain affected by Alzheimer's is dissected and examined, there are many signs of high levels of oxidative stress. Clumped neurons (nerve cells) and a substance called "beta-amyloid," both found abundantly in the brains of Alzheimer's patients, are thought to be the result of excess free radicals. We don't know for sure whether the excess free radicals are a cause or an effect of the disease, but we do know that neurons can be badly damaged by them.

The delicate tissues of the brain are protected by the blood-brain barrier. This barrier lines the blood vessels that carry oxygen-rich blood through the brain, and it won't allow any potentially harmful substances through. Antioxidants, however, can pass freely through the blood-brain barrier to affect the level of oxidative stress in the neurons. It has been found in studies of animals that vitamin E protects the neurons against oxidative damage and delays beta-amyloid-induced memory loss. And in a clinical trial of the use of vitamin E in Alzheimer's disease patients, 2,000 IUs (international units) of vitamin E a day slowed functional deterioration and delayed the necessity for placement in a nursing home. Another trial using vitamin E, this one designed to examine whether this nutrient can delay or prevent a diagnosis of Alzheimer's in older people with mild dementia, is now under way.

In *As You Like It*, William Shakespeare describes the seven ages of man. Of the last age, he writes: "Last scene of all, that ends this strange eventful history is second childishness and mere oblivion." As we learn more about aging, we find that this "second childishness" is not inevitable. Many illustrious minds have worked brilliantly into old age. George Bernard Shaw, for example, died at the age of ninety-four, having written several plays while in his nineties. I can't tell you for sure what Shaw ate during his lifetime, but the same dietary advice that helps to prevent heart disease and cancer is also likely to protect against age-related dementia.

Common Denominators

The general process of aging, as well as diseases such as cataracts, osteoporosis, and dementia, all appear to be dependent on genetic and nutritional factors with common themes. Once we sort through the complex thickets of genetics, we find that these common denominators—among them excess oxidation, and diets mismatched with genes—will respond well to the same plant-based diet rich in antioxidants. Adding supplemental antioxidants such as vitamin E, alpha-lipoic acid, and lutein to the diet can only help to prevent the onset of age-related diseases and premature aging.

YOUR GENES AND FOODS: YESTERDAY, TODAY, AND TOMORROW

14

Gene-Diet Imbalance and Damage to DNA

A baby in the womb doesn't really eat, but it is in perfect balance with its mother's genes and nutrition. A shared blood supply connects mother and fetus, and the nutrients needed by the baby are simply taken from the mother. If she is poorly nourished and has low stores of calcium, the baby will take calcium anyway to help to build its bones. Only starvation, which drastically alters the chemistry of the blood, can threaten the survival of the baby. Most babies have had perfect nutrition provided by a reasonably nourished mother, and, miraculously, most are perfect when they are born.

Despite the baby's preferential removal of nutrients from the mother, under extreme conditions such as starvation, the results of maternal malnutrition can be disastrous for the baby's development. At the very least, the baby will be small for the time it spent in the uterus. At worst, it could have birth defects such as spina bifida (a failure of the spine to fuse), due to a deficiency of the vitamin folic acid. If the mother is overnourished and diabetic during the pregnancy, the baby will sense the high levels of circulating growth factors, such as insulin, insulinlike growth factors, and growth hormone, in the mother and will grow large. This can result in the need for surgical deliveries, and in underdeveloped lands can lead to birth trauma and death during childbirth. Strong hormones taken during pregnancy, such as diethylstilbestrol, taken for nausea in the 1950s, can program infants to develop vaginal cancer in their twenties. Some researchers believe that malnutrition in the uterus somehow sets up a situation in which obesity is promoted during adulthood, but this has not been proved. So while nature has provided a number of fail-safe systems to guarantee the reproduction of our species, evidence of gene-diet imbalance can be reflected in the unborn child and can affect gene activity later in life.

Balanced Nutrition in Early Life

After the shock of entering the world is over, the baby suckles at its mother's breasts. Once again, the baby is in near perfect balance with nature and doesn't need to do much other than suckle. When the baby's stomach fills with breast milk, it stops suckling. The breast makes milk in direct response to the stimulation of the nipple, which results from suckling, so that the amount of milk made and the amount the child needs are roughly in balance. Breast-fed babies don't get fat, because their food supply is in close association with the system in their brains that controls the amount of food they eat. Their mother's breast also determines the chemical balance of the food they eat, and the composition of breast milk is genetically determined so that it, too, is in balance with the baby.

After the Breast

As soon as the baby stops suckling, all bets are off. Nutritional balance is disrupted. In those African societies that subsist on cassava fruit, the babies who are given to adoptive aunts at one year of age develop a disease called "kwashiorkor." Kwashiorkor means, literally, "separated from the breast" in Swahili, and as a result of the imbalance of the diet, which is comprised of carbohydrates with no protein, the babies develop protein and energy malnutrition. Their legs and livers swell. Their skin turns a light color due to a deficiency of the amino acid tyrosine, which is needed to make the melanin that darkens their skin. Ultimately, the immune systems of these children fail and they die of infectious diseases

Around the world the introduction of baby formula has had a long and checkered history. It has proved quite difficult to match the nutrient composition of formula with babies' nutrient needs. In one famous case a company removed the sodium from their formulas to try to prevent high blood pressure from developing later in life. A number of babies became seriously ill, and the formula was pulled off the market. Early introduction of cow's milk can also lead to problems, since cow's milk is designed for cows, not humans, and has a very different chemical composition from human milk. The early introduction of solid foods leads to abnormal weight gain in many infants, and there are some studies suggesting that this early overnutrition may enhance the infants' tendency to become overweight later in life.

Eating When You're Not Hungry

As soon as we begin to make our own food choices, we gravitate toward foods that are tasty and convenient. We begin to eat not out of hunger but because of a schedule or a social situation. Sometimes we eat because of boredom, loneliness, or sadness. The urge to eat for these reasons often overpowers the signals that say we've had enough.

Children will almost always choose an ice cream cone over a plate of steamed vegetables. In one famous psychology experiment, a group of overweight adults ate when the clock struck noon, whether they were hungry or not—and despite the fact that the real time was eleven o'clock.

In a different, naturally occurring experiment, a residence for the elderly in a Los Angeles suburb tried to improve their facility by putting a refrigerator filled with snacks in each resident's room. After a few months the refrigerators were pulled out of the rooms since the elderly residents were beginning to gain too much body fat. Whenever they were bored, they went to the refrigerator and ate something. Their hunger-control mechanisms were completely overwhelmed by their desire for foods as entertainment—a clear example of mind over matter

Eating Is Not Dining Anymore

Over the last twenty years, our lives have become more rushed than ever before. The labor-saving devices meant to reduce our workload have instead raised expectations, shortened deadlines, and compressed time lines, leaving little time for real relaxation. Even eating, which can be a pleasure-filled and leisurely process, has become rushed. Meals consist of a flurry of shoveling, chewing, and swallowing, interspersed here and there with a few glances up from the plate. Our high-stress lifestyles have brought us to this point, where we feed like animals at a trough. The food industry even recently developed a push-up omelet you could eat with one hand while driving. When we rush to ingest food without fully experiencing its textures and tastes, we eat a good deal more, and it is stressful to the body to have to continually deal with excess calories.

Tastes Great, Less Filling

Why is it that eating gets out of hand so easily when we are faced with endless quantities of high-fat, high-sugar snack foods? It's because they taste great and they're less filling. The food industry is constantly trying to find just the levels of sweetness, bitterness, saltiness, and sourness that will make their products irresistible. A sweet taste is increasingly pleasant as it becomes sweeter, until it crosses the threshold into too sweet. Similarly, salty, bitter, and sour tastes can be pleasant at one level and unpleasant at another.

The pattern of food choices and the selection of pleasant food tastes are formed as learned responses early in life. Our perception of what tastes good differs from culture to culture because of differences in the food supply. In some parts of China, for example, the taste of bitter melon is considered pleasant, while the average American would not enjoy it. One taste that is extremely abundant in the American food supply is sweet, and we seek sweetness out as we make our food choices. Corn sugar, with its pancake-syruplike taste, is the most commonly used sweetener in American colas. In other countries, such as Mexico, colas are made with table sugar (sucrose) and taste different than American colas.

The Battle for Your Taste Buds

It's natural for us to seek out pleasant, sweet tastes. Our genes were originally programmed to seek out these tastes in fruits and vegetables.

Cultural evolution has given rise to the development of methods to concentrate sugars and to develop artificial sweeteners that are much sweeter than any natural sugar. Our genetic preference for sweetness has not changed, and the sweet tastes we experience when we drink a soda or eat candy are far more concentrated than those offered by fresh fruit. Artificial sweeteners are more concentrated still. Now, our taste buds expect that intensified sweetness. When someone pairs a piece of cheesecake with coffee that has a packet of artificial sweetener stirred in, it is usually because she has found that the artificial sweetener is sweeter, and pleases her taste buds even more than sugar. The manufacturers of these sweeteners couldn't restrain themselves. They had to add enough artificial sweetener to give them the sweetness edge over sugar.

This kind of competition goes on in every food category. If you are making snack chips and your competitor amplifies the taste by adding more salt or more oil, a refusal to add more to your product could mean reduced sales. The taste buds of American consumers have been thoroughly adulterated by intensified tastes, and so the new evolutionary pressure in the grocery store is a battle to offer the most flavor without overdoing it.

The Science of Taste Modification

Food manufacturers have raised taste modification to a high level of science. There are nutritional scientists who specialize in taste research, many of whom work for the food industry. There are some indications that tastes vary in different ethnic groups, and among individuals there are inherited differences in the ability to taste certain test chemicals. Food manufacturers even target specific regions in the United States so that the same brand of cracker in the western United States will taste different from the one sold in the Deep South. As more foods are exported to Asia, the differences in taste that are prevalent will affect food processing for those regions. However, as with the whole human genome, the commonalities overwhelm the differences. Sugar and fat added to foods will increase sales almost anywhere in the world.

This battle for your taste buds has also resulted in the removal of most of the fiber that naturally occurs in plant foods. Fiber is bulky and filling, and processing it out enables consumers to eat more of a product at a sitting, so that the manufacturer can sell more of it.

The Enlarging American Plate

The typical American dinner plate has increased in size from ten inches to fourteen inches in diameter over the last twenty years. Why would restaurants want to serve more food to their customers? Wouldn't it be more profitable to give them high-fiber foods in smaller portions? No, because food is the least expensive item in restaurants. The major costs in a restaurant are labor, paid out to those who prepare and serve the meals. These costs are fixed. You can't cut your chef in half when attendance at your restaurant drops. Restaurants serve large volumes of food to give customers the idea that they are getting a good deal, and these jumbo-size portions are what American consumers have come to expect when dining out. Only the most upscale restaurants serve nouvelle cuisine, displaying an exquisite tidbit in the center of a dish and surrounding it with multi-colored sauces that radiate to the edges of the plate.

Dopamine and Food "Addictions"

It has long been accepted that alcoholism and drug addiction have some basis in genetics. While there are no withdrawal reactions when you stop eating snack foods, there are clearly addictive aspects to many food habits. It's a pleasurable experience to warm your body when it's cold, or to cool it when it's warm; there is, of course, much pleasure in the process of reproduction, and there is pleasure involved in eating. After all, nature intended for you to repeat your eating behaviors to remain well nourished. On finding and eating a good fruit or vegetable, pleasure reinforced the ancient hunter-gatherer to expend the energy needed to find that food again.

There is genetic variation in the brain's pleasure center. A neurotransmitter chemical called "dopamine," found throughout the nervous system, is instrumental in creating feelings of satisfaction and enjoyment. It is thought to be involved in most addictions, including those to drugs, alcohol, and tobacco. A genetic variation in the dopamine receptor (the brain protein that detects the dopamine signal) has been found to be present in about 30 percent of the general population, and in 70 percent of obese individuals who are also addicted to alcohol, drugs, or tobacco. This variation reduces the number of dopamine receptors in the brain by about 30 percent, so that less dopamine can click into receptor sites to trigger feelings of pleasure. One widely accepted theory relating to dopamine and addiction that is being tested is called "reward-deficiency syndrome." According to this theory, fewer dopamine receptors mean that more foods, tobacco, alcohol, or drugs are needed to bring on feelings of well-being by increasing the amounts of dopamine and other pleasure signals to this part of the brain.

Serotonin, the Pleasure Hormone

Another well-studied system involves serotonin, a pleasure-producing neurotransmitter. Serotonin is made from an amino acid, tryptophan, but the tryptophan must get into the brain to work. Tryptophan is transported into the brain across what is called the "blood-brain barrier." This barrier is actually a membrane made up of thin tissues dotted with specialized proteins. These proteins shuttle drugs and amino acids from the brain blood vessels into the fluid surrounding the brain tissue (the cerebrospinal fluid).

When you eat carbohydrates your insulin levels increase. This, in turn, increases the transport of tryptophan into the brain. So there is a grain of truth in carbohydrate craving. For carbohydrate cravers there is a strong food-mood connection. Their moods are also often affected by the amount of light in the environment. The pineal gland in the brain, which evolved from the so-called third eye in birds, responds to light-dark cycles so that there is more serotonin made during daylight hours. Light directly stimulates nerve tracts from the eye to the pineal gland. When daylight hours become shorter during certain times of the year, serotonin levels drop, causing SAD, or seasonal affective disorder. Obesity and poor eating habits often combine to worsen seasonal depression in patients with carbohydrate craving. Losing weight and improving eating habits can sometimes help to lessen these symptoms.

All of the systems discussed above work within the deep parts of the brain that deal with instinctive behaviors. Surrounding those parts are the higher-thinking areas, found in the cerebral cortex. These are the parts of the brain that enable us to worry, ponder, and stress out. The higher-thinking centers can override the lower centers, rubbing out our instinctive knowledge of what our bodies really need.

Trigger Foods and Stress

In my work with overweight individuals over the past twenty years, I have accumulated a good deal of knowledge about which foods people use for purposes other than hunger, such as stress reduction. I call these foods "trigger foods," since research has connected these food cravings with particular stress factors and the adrenal-gland hormone signals that result from stress. Many people forget to eat for much of their busy day and then eat these trigger foods as they try to relax.

The urge to eat more of a readily available, tasty food is natural, but the availability of endless quantities of great-tasting foods is decidedly not. It is thought that a Stone Age human would eat several pounds of food at a single meal if he came upon a dead carcass. The instinctive signals to keep eating as long as food is available are very strong. Let's face it: Ancient humans didn't know where their next meal was coming from, but we do. We're not going to run out of food, so we have to know when to stop eating it.

Binge-Eating Disorder

What motivates binge eating? A major motivation is the pleasurable signals sent to the brain as you fill up with food. At the same time, your brain is dealing with stressful signals, originally developed to enable you to flee from a predator or to heighten your senses in moments of danger. This made sense in ancient times, when a predator could attack you as you hunted or gathered your day's fare, but today's version of this stress is found in the context of social situations that are much more complex. Stressful stimuli often linger for long periods of time or never really go away at all, causing unrelenting anxiety. The pleasure signals triggered by eating certain foods can counteract this stress and its unpleasant psychological and physical consequences.

Binge eating is simply eating without end or until the box or bag of trigger food is empty. It is estimated that up to 25 percent of all obese individuals engage in binge eating. A lot of binge eating occurs at night, when the stresses of the day come back to haunt us. You don't have to go any farther than your kitchen to saturate your pleasure center with whatever happens to be available. The open refrigerator and pantry door become objects of contemplation for the nighttime binge eater.

Binge-eating disorders, including night snacking, are estimated to affect about one fourth of obese individuals.

A great deal has been learned about the feedback mechanisms controlling our food-seeking and eating behaviors, all of which evolved in a very different environment from the one we live in today. When diet books ask people to restrict their food intake, they are asking them to perform an unnatural act. We are wired to seek out pleasant-tasting foods and to eat them when we find them. Modern agribusiness and modern food processing have bypassed our natural mechanisms for controlling food intake and body weight.

Overeating and the Risk of Diabetes, Heart Disease, and Cancer

Eating at the trough will do more than increase your weight. Over-consumption of high-calorie foods sends signals throughout your body that turn on cell division. Increased cell division is the first step toward the formation of cancerous growths, and plays a role in clogging arteries and piling on extra pounds that can predispose you to diabetes. As cells divide, free-radical production is increased, possibly leading to DNA damage and cancer formation. This is especially true when the diet is high in calories but lacks antioxidant nutrients. When you provide your cells with excess calories without the phytochemicals that nature originally packaged with them, you set the stage for tumor development.

It has been estimated that one in two men and one in three women over fifty years of age will be diagnosed with cancer in the next few decades. With modern methods of diagnosis, most of these cancers will be small and treatable. More energy will be focused on finding ways to prevent the cancer from recurring. Evidence has shown that when women with breast cancer lose weight after the diagnosis, their prognoses are improved more than those of women who gain weight.

What You Can Learn from a Rat

Our laboratory rats also eat at the trough—literally. They are provided with all the pellets they can eat. By two years of age, they are uniformly obese and have impaired immune function and cancer. When we put these animals on a diet, we reduce the incidence of cancer, improve immune function, and extend life span. When we give these rats a bland, monotonous diet, they are better able to control their body weight. They eat when hungry, and stop when they are full.

If we feed rats what we call a "cafeteria diet," made up of a variety of snack foods such as peanut butter, chocolate, cookies, and pepperoni, they become as obese as animals with severe forms of genetic obesity. In people, variety can also stimulate overeating. In a study by Dr. Susan Roberts of Tufts University, it was found that increasing variety within any category of foods—with the exception of vegetables and fruits—caused weight gain. Increasing the variety of vegetables was associated with a decrease in body weight, and increasing the variety of fruits eaten had no net effect on body weight.

Our genetics are similar enough to those of rats that the basic principles of energy balance and food intake apply to both species. Man and mouse alike must follow the first law of thermodynamics: Energy taken in must equal energy out and energy stored. In the absence of increased physical activity, if we eat more food energy, that energy will be stored as fat.

Fat Cells and Your Set-Point

The body's fat cells are not passive; they also send feedback signals to the brain to reduce food intake and increase physical activity. This is where the idea of a genetic set-point gains scientific credibility. In a given set of circumstances, genetics determine an individual's level of body fat and the distribution of that body fat. In Denmark during World War II, twins were separated and raised in different homes. Many years later they were brought together and photographed. Despite having been raised in different home environments, their body fat, body weight, and the pattern of fat deposits in their bodies were remarkably similar.

Fat and muscle patterns are genetically determined to some extent, but the amount of fat and muscle depend on the results of the behaviors of individuals in terms of food intake and exercise. The shocking fact that one of two Americans is overweight is testimony to the imbalance of genes and diets in our society. This has resulted from a combination of individual behaviors, genetic predisposition, and the socioeconomic factors that have altered our food supply both in terms of quantity of foods and the nature of those foods by comparison with our natural food supplies thousands of years ago.

Why Women Are Fatter Than Men

Why is it that women have more body fat at a given body weight than men, even when they consume less food? Women tend to have less muscle mass than men of the same height. Muscle burns about 14 calories per pound per day, while body fat burns very few. It is typical for a woman seen in my clinic to burn 1,200 to 1,400 calories per day at rest, while her husband burns 2,000 to 2,200 calories per day while at rest. Despite eating fewer calories than her husband, she still gains weight and has a terrible time controlling her body fat.

In women fat cells in some parts of the body grow in response to female hormones. Fat is an important organ when it comes to maintaining a pregnancy and breast-feeding. In surviving hunter-gatherer cultures, women feed their babies at the breast for one to two years. Each day breast milk carries about 500 calories out of the body. To be able to store these calories, women have to develop stores of hip and thigh fat. Men don't get fat below the waist until they are older, or have elevated levels of female hormones.

However, for women, this balance of fat changes throughout life. With the onset of puberty, fat is deposited in the hips and thighs. This can take a varying amount of time from woman to woman. Some women don't fully develop their female fat until their first pregnancy. As menopause approaches the fat redistributes to the middle of the body and breast fat increases.

This redistribution of body fat is a programmed change in our genes that occurred with the evolution of menopause. Menopause is a purely human phenomenon, and now that women are living well beyond the "change of life," the genetics of menopause and aging has to be accounted for in postmenopausal women who want to balance genes with diet.

Men have changes in hormones with aging, in what has recently been termed "andropause." As he ages a man's muscle mass decreases, his male hormone levels drop, and his female hormones may increase slightly. A little pouch of fat develops below his belt in response to increased levels of female hormones.

The Big Picture

Eating at the trough, the final aberration in our nutritional environment, has served to unbalance our diet and our genes. It cannot be seen in isolation, but must be considered in the context of underactivity, a narrowed and monotonous diet, reduced fiber intake, reduced intake of health-giving substances from plant foods, and increased intakes of refined sugar and added, processed vegetable oils. The imbalance of this diet and our genes cannot be solved by simply taking a multivitamin. While in many societies vitamin deficiencies result from monotonous diets, the advent, in the 1950s, of fortified foods such as milk fortified with vitamin A and D and vitamin-fortified cereals have made obvious vitamin deficiencies uncommon in American society. Certain genes that evolved in another long-ago era have programmed our bodies to expect a diverse array of plant foods that we no longer eat. This imbalance will turn out to play a key role in promoting chronic diseases, including heart disease and cancer, in genetically susceptible individuals.

15

Cultural Evolution and the Loss of Eden

The foods that end up in our supermarkets and on our dining tables are a product of 2 million years of human evolution. At some point in history, the paths of biological and cultural evolution began to diverge, and since that time we have been industriously creating an environment with which our biology is ill-prepared to coexist.

This chapter will be devoted to tracing the course of the nutritional cultural evolution that created an imbalance between genes and nutrients. Knowing where we came from allows us to understand what the body needs in order to return to a state of balance and health.

A Brief Early History of Humans on Earth

Life began on earth several billion years ago, and dinosaurs died out 65 million years ago. About 10 million years ago, our prehuman ancestors began to walk upright, having evolved enough to be distinguishable from our closest relatives, gorillas and chimpanzees. Another species destined to lead to humans began walking upright in Africa 4 million years ago. And 2 million years ago there were two and possibly three prehuman species, one of which began to make crude stone axes at about this time.

By about 1.7 million years ago, *Homo erectus*—an extinct predecessor of *Homo sapiens*, the species of modern humans—was present across Africa, eating a diverse diet containing meat, plants, and insects. About a million years ago, *Homo erectus* left Africa for the first time and traveled east, to the far reaches of Asia. Archaeological digs have uncovered the remains of *Homo erectus* in China, Java, and Europe.

The modern human, or *Homo sapiens*, appeared on the scene only about 500,000 years ago, a blink in the time line of our planetary evolution. Between 130,000 and 40,000 years ago, another species arose in Europe that was not quite like *Homo erectus* or *Homo sapiens*. This species, now commonly called Neanderthal man, was very likely a different species that could not procreate successfully with *Homo sapiens*. Neanderthal man disappeared 40,000 years ago, leaving modern humans to migrate out of Africa and spread across Eurasia. A key step that most scientists believe accelerated cultural evolution to give *Homo sapiens* a leg up on all previous prehumans was the development of language. Between 100,000 and 50,000 years ago, the development of the voice box or a change in brain structure may have led to the development of language, and with it the spoken word.

Mankind Explores Earth

As humans spread across the globe, they encountered a wide variety of environmental conditions and indigenous foods. Humans from Africa reached Siberia about twenty thousand years ago, and crossed into Alaska and the North American continent only twelve thousand years ago. In the process of finding ways to subsist and thrive in these diverse settings, their cultural evolution progressed at a reasonable pace. Their genes may have had to make some slight adaptations, but until the advent of modern agriculture and processed foods, they remained more or less in balance with their surroundings and the foods they ate.

One Big, Happy Family?

Before humans began their migration out of Africa, they lived there in a sort of Garden of Eden—a highly biodiverse environment that molded human DNA in such a way as to allow the species as a whole to survive and flourish. A recent article in the journal *Science*, by Dr. Kelly Owens and Dr. Mary Claire King, both scientists at the University of Washington in Seattle, points out that because of our common origins in this Garden of Eden, the entire concept of race, with its enormous impact on world politics and human relationships, is a faulty one—that the idea that human history is the story of different races is biologically flawed. According to Drs. Owens and King, all important variations in the human genetic code happened before humans migrated out of Africa and evolved into what we now know as the different races. In populations made up of people who all share the same skin color and heritage, as well as in the ethnic melting pot of the modern American city, the genome of each person contains about 85 percent of all possible variations in the human gene pool.

Scientific evidence supports their theory. Superficial traits of skin color and facial features probably reflect the influences of various climates on an already established human genome. The most obvious differences among races are those of skin and hair color. Skin and hair color appear to vary because of a small variation in one type of hormone receptor. In fair-skinned individuals there is a variation in a receptor for the hormone that stimulates the darkening of skin (the melanocyte-stimulating hormone). It appears that the simple absence of this variation is what causes skin to be dark rather than light in Africans and others who do not sunburn easily. At some point in history, Caucasian skin evolved from African skin because of this mutation in the gene that codes for the melanocyte-stimulating hormone receptor.

Pop's Y Chromosomes
and Mom's Mitochondria

Some of the variations in the Y chromosome, which is carried only by men, lend further support to Drs. King and Owens's ideas. Other support comes from variations in the DNA carried on subcellular (smaller than a cell) structures called "mitochondria," which contain their own DNA and are handed down through the mother's genetic endowment to her offspring. Let's look more closely at this.

When an egg cell is fertilized, it accepts DNA from the nucleus of the sperm cell, and this is the father's contribution to the child's genetic makeup. The mother's contribution comes from the egg cell's cytoplasm, the watery matter that surrounds the nucleus and contains the mitochondria and other important components of the cell. The mitochondria act as submicroscopic energy generators that fuel cellular activity. Mitochondria are thought to be some type of primitive bacteria that during evolution somehow became incorporated, with their own DNA, into primitive cells. This addition endowed cells with the ability to produce energy by "burning" fuel sources such as carbohydrates and fats with the help of oxygen, yielding water and carbon dioxide as end products.

Sons inherit a Y chromosome from their fathers and an X chromosome from their mothers. The Y chromosome is what confers maleness; without it, the child will be a girl, having inherited an X chromosome from each parent.

High Priests and Invading Armies

By examining areas of variation in DNA sequences on Y chromosomes, it is possible to trace male migrations, while looking at the DNA of mitochondria has enabled us to separately trace the migration of women. Genetic studies of the Y chromosome have confirmed the distinctive identity of the Cohanim, a Jewish tribe from which priests were descended in the era of the temple in Jerusalem. This tradition is still passed down from father to sons. Although there is no longer an actual priesthood, today, in synogogues, these men recite special prayers on behalf of the whole congregation. Among different groups of Jews from many countries throughout the world, the male Cohanim carry the same unique gene on their Y chromosome. At the same time, studies of mitochondrial DNA in different countries around the world have demonstrated that women were conquered and taken prisoner by invading armies, leading to a greater admixture of genetic material from women than from men. The men of conquered tribes were killed in various parts of the world, and so their Y chromosomes were not handed down to succeeding generations, while their wives' mitochondrial DNA survived.

Genetic Evidence of a Lost Tribe in Africa

Groups such as the Ashkenazi Jews of Eastern Europe, who wandered far from their origins in the Middle East, have mitochondrial DNA that is more genetically similar to other populations in the Middle East and in North Africa than to other Eastern Europeans—a good indication that they originated in the Middle East. Genetic evidence also supports the oral tradition that the Lemba, a Bantu-speaking people in southern Africa, evolved from Jews who migrated from the Middle East to Yemen 2,700 years ago and to southern Africa 2,000 to 2,400 years ago. Over 50 percent of the Y chromosomes among the Lemba carry genes that are common in Jewish populations but are absent in their African neighbors.

Moving Up the Nile River

All of this evidence demonstrates the power of genetics to trace human history. The analysis of the DNA found in the mitochondria of African tribes along the Nile River is consistent with a northward migration pattern into Lower Egypt. This DNA evidence establishes the origins of man in Africa, and supports the central idea of this book that man once lived in a rich and biodiverse environment in subtropical Africa in ancient times. Further research on this DNA found that most human genetic variation antedates the migration of man out of Africa. The DNA of the tribes from Africa included 85 percent of the variation we observe in modern populations throughout the world today. If DNA is examined from any group around the world today, the same degree of variability among the DNA of individuals is observed. So the differences in our individual DNA that enable us to break down different chemicals in our environment or make us susceptible to chronic disease are very ancient genes that were already very different among humans evolving in the Gardens of Eden somewhere in Africa. This body of work also demonstrates that the genes that determine our optimal diet evolved independent of race, and reflect the biodiverse diet consumed by humans in Africa millions of years ago.

Prescription Drugs,
Plant Foods, and Genes

Different races have some differences in the genes that code for the enzymes that carry out the breakdown of a variety of prescription drugs. Drug companies are searching for the individual genes that enable medications to be easily tolerated by some people but cause serious side effects in others. These genes are in the same families that evolved to handle the chemicals found in plant foods such as fruits and vegetables. After all, there were no drugs fifty thousand years ago. The risks for cancer, heart disease, and diabetes vary considerably between ethnic groups—and only some of the differences can be accounted for by differences in racial origin. Asians migrating to the United States markedly increase their risks of these chronic diseases within one generation, but some differences in incidence compared to Caucasian populations living in the United States persist. Are these differences in chronic-disease risk genetically based, or are they dependent on diet and lifestyle? We don't yet have the knowledge to answer that question with 100 percent certainty, but most likely it is a combination of the two.

Genes and environment appear to interact to modulate the risk of disease in any individual. Since ancient humans left Africa, enough time has elapsed that subtle differences in the genome, which are important in translating the effects of diet on the development of chronic diseases and aging, have evolved. Recognizing the differences among individuals, regardless of ethnic origin, is an important step toward understanding why the right diet for your genes may reduce the risk of developing a chronic disease.

The Coevolution of Animal and Plant Life

What have humans been eating since their first days in the forests, mountains, and deserts of Africa? For most of the 7 million years of prehuman and human existence, we were hunter-gatherers, subsisting on wild animals and plants. While there are famous paintings in French caves of large bison, it is likely that the majority of the ancient human diet in Africa was made up of wild plants, berries, roots, and leaves, with some animal protein, including that of insects. Humans let their taste buds guide them to the nutritious foods that were abundant enough to provide adequate protein and calories.

Taste and smell are marvels of nature that permit us to sensitively interact with our environment and interpret the presence or absence of tiny amounts of molecules. People who lose their sense of smell can no longer taste, and the improved tastes of warm foods are partially related to the experience of the smell of the foods. This system is one of the most important throughout nature. A wild moth can smell, from a few miles away, a few molecules of an attractant chemical for mating called a pheromone. Many fish species see poorly but depend on smell for finding prey. For humans, we have used these senses not only to find food but also to enjoy food.

The Modern Jungle Is a TV Commercial

Our visual and auditory senses are bombarded by advertising for this or that food, and this is how we make our food choices today. Even commercially available whole foods, such as fruits and vegetables, have in some cases been bred to be bland, dull, and starchy because of consumer preferences for certain textures and tastes and the need to transport produce to market without significant damage occurring in transit. While our taste preferences have been used by advertisers to entice us away from our gene-diet balance, the pleasure of eating is an inherited trait that we should not lose.

Before civilization changed our methods for hunting down and gathering nourishment, humans relied on their senses to help them choose which plant foods to eat. Today most people's taste buds have been corrupted by a steady diet of highly processed foods, with their added sugar, hidden fats and oils, and artificial flavorings and colorings. The switch back to our culinary roots will require major adjustments in our perception of what is most delicious, and will involve efforts to obtain whole foods that are grown in traditional ways.

Man Disrupts the Gardens of Eden

In the ancient African Gardens of Eden (there was probably more than one), a human tribe's selections of which plants to eat had a powerful influence on which plants survived and which died out. Thousands of years ago, if one berry was in competition with another for the attention of hungry hunter-gatherers, it grew to a larger size or developed a sweeter taste. All of the instinctive mechanisms that go into the hunter-gatherer's food choices and food-seeking behaviors are geared to the reality that he or she must eat pounds of a biodiverse array of foods that contain all of the beneficial chemicals, calories, fat, minerals, and vitamins necessary for survival. This diet is far more diverse than the "basic four food groups" I learned about in medical school, or even the more recently developed USDA food pyramid. While modern agriculture, food processing, and marketing have provided us with plentiful food supplies, we have lost the biodiversity of ancient diets.

Primitive humans were also attracted to plant foods by their bright colors, the ratio of edible to inedible material, taste, and texture. In each instance humans were one of many animals influencing plant genetics through selection. Obviously, plants don't sit around planning out their exact strategy for attracting animals to feed on them. Instead, they play a time-consuming game of trial and error, with the berries that are the right size and taste winning out for selection and spread in the environment.

Over eons this sort of interaction between humans, plants, insects, and other life forms created a balance between the human diet and the environment, and to a large extent shaped our genetic makeup. Just as a fish living in the ocean must develop special mechanisms to interact with that salty water, so the human body interacted with and adapted to the chemicals in foods over millions of years. We developed specific tactics for detoxifying poisons, conserving rare elements of the diet, and promoting the proper balance of nutrients. It is these mechanisms and their imbalance with our modern diet, which has developed in only the past century, that explains much of the current epidemic of chronic diseases.

The Emergence of Agriculture

In those parts of the world endowed with richly biodiverse environments, such as California, the hunter-gatherer lifestyle persisted until European colonizers came on the scene within the last six hundred years. With a large desert to the east and the ocean to the west, California was a virtual island, occupied by about a hundred native Indian tribes speaking a hundred languages. Their primary source of protein was the acorn of the wild oak tree, which was never domesticated. They ate a variety of different plants and some fish and shellfish from the ocean. The rich Mediterranean environment of California, with its mountains and valleys, provided the perfect setting for the growth of a biodiverse diet. Even today, 50 percent of the U.S. supply of fruits and vegetables is grown in California soil. This includes over 250 varieties, 70 of which are grown solely in California. Although there is evidence that the California Native Americans knew about farming from their trade contacts with Native Americans in Arizona, they did not adopt an agricultural lifestyle. They didn't have to farm to feed themselves. The California climate exists in a few other places on earth, including the Fertile Crescent in the Middle East, a small area of Chile, the Argentine pampas, parts of Australia, and parts of the Cape of South Africa.

The Ice Age and Mutated Plant Foods

Agriculture arose at the end of the second Ice Age in the Fertile Crescent, which extended across modern Iraq and Iran. At that particular time—about ten thousand years ago—wild wheat mutated to retain its seed on its stalk rather than scatter it to the wind as other strains did. This strain was harvested and eaten by the first farmers, and agriculture was born. These farmers continued to gather and hunt while supplementing their biodiverse food supply with a few easily grown crops.

Humans began to shape natural selection by taking advantage of natural mutations that favored using particular crops as food. The single genetic mutation that caused the seeds of wild wheat to remain on the stalk would have been a lethal mutation in the absence of humans, since the plant needed to scatter its seeds to reproduce. Humans intervened, however, and those mutant plants with retained seeds were the ones humans selected to harvest and plant to grow more wheat. Similarly, from over 150 other edible pea species, humans chose to grow peas that stayed in the pod.

Other mutations selected by humans included a thin seed coat and self-fertilization. The thin seed coat favored easy germination in tilled and watered soil. The other mutation, self-fertilization, was chosen because the characteristics that made the crops easy to plant and harvest would be lost if the plants were bred with pollen from wild strains.

Animal domestication also happened in a cooperative manner. People began to keep wild animals penned up for their use, but animals also began to find that living near people had its advantages.

Why did agriculture start in the Fertile Crescent? Ten thousand years ago the climate conditions were suitable, and the area had a large number of large-seeded grass species that could give rise to wheat and barley seed mutants that would retain their grain and be easy to harvest. As early as 8500 B.C., sickles had been invented in this part of the world to harvest domesticated wheat. Prior to the domestication of animals, the only way to transport goods was on the backs of humans; goats and sheep could carry goods over long distances, and even provided fertilizer in exchange for their room and board. This advance in transportation helped agriculture to slowly spread through the Middle East and into Greece about 6000 B.C.

Plant and Crop Domestication

Over time, domesticated crops and animals were introduced to new areas, and in each new area additional species were domesticated. The fruits of these labors often made their way back to the place from which the original domesticated plants and animals had come. Slowly, agriculture spread throughout Eurasia. About 7000 B.C. sesame, eggplant, and humped cattle were domesticated in India. In about 6000 B.C. sycamores, figs, donkeys, and cats were domesticated in Egypt. About 4000 B.C. olive trees were domesticated for the oil found in their fruits, and the domestication of other fruit trees that could be grown from either seeds or cuttings, such as dates, pomegranates, and grapes, followed. Between 6000 B.C. and 3500 B.C., poppies and oats were domesticated in Europe.

The next agricultural phase in Europe was the cultivation of trees that must be grown by grafting, such as apple, pear, plum, and cherry. At around the same time, wild plants such as radishes, rye, turnips, beets, leeks, and lettuce that had initially established themselves as weeds were domesticated. By the time of the Roman Empire, many of today's leading crops were domesticated. After 1500 the vast fertile plains of the New World brought great enrichment to the world's food supply.

The domestication of crops and livestock sprang up independently in some parts of the world. This suggests that, given enough time, humans would have eventually domesticated plants and animals in many areas of the world even if the practice had not migrated from one land to the next. For example, there is evidence that in China, rice, millet, and pigs were domesticated independent of domestication elsewhere around 6500 B.C. In about 3500 B.C., South Americans domesticated potatoes, manioc, guinea pigs, and llamas. In Mesoamerica, independent of developments in South America, corn, beans, squash, and turkeys were domesticated around 3500 B.C. Sunflowers and goosefoot plants, but no animals, were domesticated by Native Americans in the eastern United States about 2500 B.C. The corn, beans, squash, and turkeys found by explorers landing in North America were brought there from Mesoamerica. In tropical West Africa African yams and oil palm were domesticated about 3000 B.C.

From Discovery of a
New World to Fusion Cuisine

A major change in the human food supply came along with the discovery of the Americas in 1492 by Christopher Columbus. Prior to 1492 people ate much the same food throughout Europe, but by 1600 there was an active exchange of foods across the seas. Old World crops were introduced to Mexico and Peru to support the Spanish lifestyle. The French, Italian, and Spanish cuisines you are familiar with would not exist without New World spices, fruits, and vegetables, which were taken to Europe mostly on Spanish ships. Szechuan Chinese food, for example, would not be Szechuan if chili peppers had not been brought from South America before 1700.

The melding of the Old and New Worlds brought about a revolution in the human diet, and a second food revolution is occurring now with the introduction of a global fusion of various cuisines. California is a leader in this movement; where else would chefs dream up a dish like Thai chicken pizza?

Early American Foods

Soon after the English moved into the eastern part of North America, they began to combine European crops with northeastern American crops. From the Indians the New Englanders learned how to clear land of trees and grow, with the aid of fish fertilizer, corn, beans, pumpkins, white potatoes, and squash. In fact, history suggests that the settlers were so inept at farming when they arrived that they would have starved to death without the Indians' help—hence the Thanksgiving story.

New Englanders took over cleared farmland after huge numbers of Indians died of smallpox. European livestock thrived in New England, especially pigs. One of the earliest American exports was barrels of pork. Colonists exported horses to the West Indies, and brought in turnip, carrot, buckwheat, pea, parsnip, wheat, barley, and oat seeds.

The Midwest Takes Over

The 1800s in America saw the westward migration and tremendous expansion of agriculture. In 1800 there were 450,000 American farms. By 1850 there were 1.5 million. Most of the early western settlers had farmed on the East Coast and had the necessary skills to work the land. The country was empty, land was cheap or free, and the law left them alone. The invention of the machines that began to mechanize harvesting and planting greatly enriched American agricultural practices, and this heyday of farming continued until about 1850. Settlers on the Great Plains of the Midwest grew corn, which became the quintessential American crop and a major export to European countries, where it began to replace other grains. By World War II the United States produced enough food to feed the world, largely due to the development in 1940 of hybrid corn varieties that increased greatly the output of corn per acre. In fact, the impact of corn is still felt in our American diets today as we have corn sugar, corn oil, and corn-fed beef. We are even using ethanol from corn in gasoline, but most of the crop is being fed to domesticated animals for edible meat production.

After World War II we paid our farmers not to plant as part of the farm price-support system made more critical by the great surpluses that would otherwise have depressed the price of farm crops. Today, agribusiness in America has unprecedented production capabilities. Recently we gave away $500 million worth of wheat to Russia without any negative impact on our farm economy.

The USDA Pyramid: Horse,
Camel, or Prescription for Obesity?

Our genes caused us to crave sweet and fat tastes, and our every dream came true in the 1950s. Our diets were like the gas-guzzling cars of the 1960s. These cars were fast, smooth, and powerful, but they polluted the environment. Our diets by the 1980s were the best modern man could devise to match our American tastes as articulated by Madison Avenue, but they proved to be less than optimal for our health.

The USDA pyramid was developed in the 1980s with the laudable aim of teaching the American public to eat in a healthier fashion. Unfortunately, the result was the typical camel that emerges when a horse is designed by a committee. The base of the pyramid consists of refined carbohydrates such as breads, cereals, rice, and pasta. These low-fiber foods are easy to eat in large portions and can contribute to weight gain. Vegetables and fruits are divided into two groups on the next level, which makes them seem less important. This was done because it was felt by some committee members that it would be wrong to combine them since fruits (in their view) tasted better than vegetables and would be overemphasized in consumers' food choices. The real problem is that people don't eat enough of either category.

A dairy group consisting of milk, yogurt, and cheeses is featured side by side with a meat, bean, and nuts group. This combination did not increase dairy consumption, as hoped by the pyramid builders who justified this division with the idea that calcium could be obtained only by eating dairy products.

Amazingly, the tip of the USDA pyramid has no foods whatsoever, just dots of oil and sugar. If you look carefully, you can see these scattered through all the levels of the pyramid with the not-so-subtle message that wherever you go in the American food supply, oil and sugar will follow you for the rest of your days. The USDA pyramid, put together by well-intentioned scientists, is, regrettably, a prescription for obesity.

One group of foods that is conspicuously absent from the USDA pyramid is the herbs and spices group. In a pyramid developed in 1997 under my leadership at the UCLA Center for Human Nutrition, these foods—which are rich in nutrients and add wonderful flavors to meals—are included at the top of the pyramid rather than oils and sugars. The "California Cuisine Pyramid" has fruits and vegetables at the base to encourage the intake of phytonutrients in foods that generally have

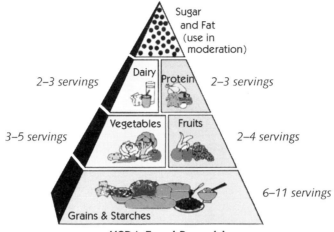

USDA Food Pyramid

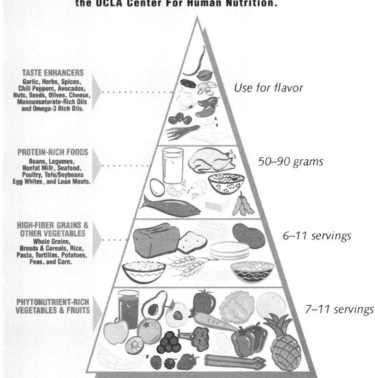

Figure 7: Comparison of USDA and California Pyramids

fewer calories per bite than refined carbohydrates. The next level up is occupied by high-fiber whole cereals and grains. The next level encourages the intake of protein in adequate amounts while avoiding extra fat and calories. The top of the pyramid adds the important dimension of taste by featuring taste enhancers such as nuts, seeds, oil, cheese, and spices rather than the drops of largely hidden oil and sugar at the top of the USDA pyramid.

While we can't turn back the clock to prehistoric Africa, when our genes were more perfectly adapted to a biodiverse plant environment, perhaps we can use our modern understanding of genetics to develop a better contemporary diet—one that is matched to our genes rather than to historical events and economics.

16

Food Evolution and Agricultural Economics

How have our current diets moved so far from what our genes expect? Tracing the path we have taken from the Garden of Eden to the present day will help us to withstand the constant barrage of advertising and the rapid comings and goings of the food fads that shape our diets.

Do you ever think about the foods you eat? Most of us don't. We assume that since humans first began to populate the earth, the balance of nutrients has been much the same as what we eat now. But if you take a few moments to think this through, you begin to realize that our ancestors probably didn't consume anything remotely similar to the processed-food diets that grace most modern tables.

America's favorite foods have a remarkably recent history. It is amazing how rapidly certain foods such as hot dogs, peanut butter, ice cream sundaes, potato chips, and doughnuts became popular. It is important to review this brief history for a couple of reasons. First, with everything you have learned so far about the evolution of foods, you can see that cultural evolution moves quickly, without regard for human biology beyond appealing to our taste buds. Second, if these foods became popular so quickly, other, healthier foods also could. The challenge to our food industry is to incorporate health into the engineering of foods, and to our government to create a level playing field in the food industry by promoting the development of healthier alternatives to our favorite foods.

The History of the Potato Chip

Thomas Jefferson brought fried potatoes to this country from France, and served them to rave reviews at a White House dinner. Then, in 1853, a restaurant customer in Saratoga Springs, New York, complained about the thickness of his fried potatoes and returned them to the cook. Supposedly, out of spite, the cook sliced some potatoes as thin as possible, fried them, and sent them back to the picky customer. To the cook's surprise the man loved them, and a popular new dish was born.

Known as "Saratoga chips," they were served primarily in restaurants until the 1890s, when William Tappendon, of Cleveland, Ohio, started the first potato chip factory in his barn. Then, in 1926, the potato chip bag was invented by Laura Scudder of California. The invention of the continuous fryer in 1929 increased production, but potato chips became more popular in 1933 with the introduction of the first waxed-paper potato chip bag providing longer shelf life for the chips. Also, you could print messages such as "You can't eat just one!," as on the famous Lay's potato chip bag. Then Pringles arrived, in a can with all the chips stacked one on top of another, perfectly shaped to fit together. In Japan this form of potato chip was regarded as quintessential American technology—a higher form of potato chip—and it continues to sell worldwide. There are carrot chips and other vegetable chips that have some color and nutrition, but they are usually made with lots of oil. The introduction of Olestra, a sucrose-polyester fat substitute, into Wow!-brand potato chips cut the calories in half, from 150 calories for 20 chips to about 75 calories for 20 chips. There were none of the side effects from eating Olestra that had been predicted by consumer groups, other than the usual amount of gastrointestinal distress we have in America now. The chips are now being enjoyed with less fat. They are not a cure for obesity, but they are not any worse than a pretzel or some popcorn.

Don't Take Away My Doughnuts!

From Homer Simpson chomping doughnuts while working at the fictional Springfield Nuclear Power Plant, to the LAPD motorcycle cop on a coffee break ordering his favorite cream-filled special, doughnuts are established as one of America's favorite foods. The great fear of every doughnut eater is that the government will figure out a way to prohibit eating these circles of fat and sweet the way they have found ways to discourage smoking cigarettes. There is probably little chance of that, but the so-called cholesterol-free doughnuts made with lots of hydrogenated vegetable oil could be improved and could provide some nutrition as well as taste.

Know where the doughnut came from? Here's the story. The doughnut arrived in America in the 1800s from Holland, where they were called "oily cakes," an appropriate but less appealing name. A sailor named Hanson Gregory took credit for the hole in the center, skewering on a ship's wheel the cakes his mother baked. The first doughnut machine was invented in 1920 in New York City by a Russian immigrant. Doughnut machines were proudly displayed, at the 1934 Chicago World's Fair, and the circles boiling in oil showed consumers what was called "the food hit of the Century of Progress." Franchising came to doughnuts after Krispy Kreme opened its first store in 1937 in Winston-Salem, North Carolina. Dunkin' Donuts opened in 1950 in Quincy, Massachusetts. America alone produces about 10 billion doughnuts a year.

Red-Hot Dachshunds and Salisbury Steaks

Nothing is more American than a hot dog at a ball game, right? Actually, the hot dog started out as a "frankfurter" from the city of Frankfurt-am-Main, Germany, in the fifteenth century, not coming to the United States until the 1800s. By 1871 a Coney Island food stand was selling "dachshund sausages" on split-bread rolls. During a cold ball game at New York's Polo Grounds around the year 1900, a vendor was losing money trying to sell ice cream and soda. He bought up all the dachshund sausages he could find and put them in hot water tanks, then hollered, "Red hot! Get your dachshunds, while they're red hot!" as he walked through the stands. A sports cartoonist named Tad Dorgan drew a picture of a talking sausage in a bun, but couldn't spell "dachshund." So he simply called them "hot dogs."

The classic novel *The Jungle* by Upton Sinclair described the conditions in a meat factory where they produced hot dogs under appalling conditions. As Americans became more health conscious, low-fat chicken, low-fat turkey, and low-fat soy hot dogs all surfaced. Except for the true hot dog gourmet, they all serve as well at the ball game or on the Fourth of July and represent ways of improving the health of a treat while maintaining the experience.

The hamburger has a similar historical origin in Germany, and during World War II they were renamed "Salisbury steaks." So-called lean burgers and turkey burgers made with dark meat can be over 40 percent fat. Very low fat soy burgers covered with relish, tomato ketchup, and a whole-wheat bun can also pull off the same trick as the soy hot dog. The franchising and mechanization of burger and French fry production by McDonald's Corporation has brought this American treat to millions around the world. The key to the standardization of the taste is the beef flavor associated with the fat in the burger and the fries. By making that taste take over, the variability in hamburger quality in restaurants was done away with at fast-food restaurants. A 50-50 soy burger, one that's half soy and half beef, maintains the taste if the full soy burger is too much for you.

Ketchup or Catsup?

"Ke-tsiap" was a pickled fish sauce from China that made its way to Malaysia, where it was known as "ketjap." Similar to soy sauce, the ketjap was brought home by English sailors in the 1600s. It was a spicy topping made from mushrooms, oysters, or unripe walnuts, and became known as "ketchup." Tomatoes were added sometime in the 1700s and the product was called "tomato ketchup" to distinguish it from the original ketchup. Variations in spelling, such as "catsup," are acceptable and come from different adaptations of the original Chinese or Malaysian ketchup. It was only in 1876, the year of the disputed election of Rutherford B. Hayes as president, that tomato ketchup was bottled and sold throughout the United States. The tremendous popularity of the tomato-based condiment overshadowed its other variations. Soon enough, the word "tomato" was no longer necessary in front of ketchup. Ketchup adds lycopene to the diet and is bioavailable, as in tomato sauces and soups, but you would have to have half a glass of ketchup to get enough, and the Federal Trade Commission stopped ketchup makers from claiming a health benefit.

There is also sugar and vinegar in ketchup, which adds to its taste appeal. While India is known for curry and China for soy sauce, America has no traditional spice of its own other than ketchup. Nonetheless, it is not a vegetable serving when you add some to French fries.

The Invention of Peanut Butter

In the 1890s, John Harvey Kellogg, who brought us breakfast cereals, ground up peanuts for his vegetarian patients and patented peanut butter. In 1904, C. H. Sumner introduced peanut butter to the masses at the St. Louis world's fair, and the Krema Products Company (still in business today) began selling peanut butter in 1908.

Modern peanut butter debuted in the early 1920s when Joseph Rosefield churned it to ensure smoothness and invented a method of making it shelf-stable so that the oil and peanut butter didn't separate. The Swift Company used Rosefield's method for its E. K. Pond peanut butter, later known as Peter Pan to baby boomers watching the Disney television show in the sixties. Peanut butter and jelly sandwiches have become emergency food for children who turn down everything else they are offered. The universal appeal of peanut butter is illustrated by the fact that the appetite controls of a mouse or rat can be overcome by feeding it peanut butter. The taste is so great, these rodents become as fat as genetically prone strains of mice and rats. Not a source of protein as much as of fat, the childhood preference for peanut butter shows up in candies, cracker sandwiches, and even as a peanut-sauce topping for Thai chicken.

Never on Sundae

Nothing is finer than a hot fudge sundae topped with whipped cream and a maraschino cherry. How did this all-American treat evolve? Iced desserts were introduced into Europe from the East. Marco Polo brought back descriptions of fruit ices from his travels in China. Italian cooks developed recipes and techniques for making both water and milk ices. In 1670 a Sicilian, Francisco Procopio, opened a café in Paris and began to sell ices and sherbets, which became so popular that by 1676 there were 250 ice makers in the French capital. Tortoni, owner of a café in late-eighteenth-century Paris, is credited with developing cream ices. In the United States ice cream was served by George Washington, Thomas

Jefferson, and Dolley Madison. Philadelphia became the hub of ice cream manufacture in the United States; the ice cream soda was invented there in 1874. The ice cream cone, portable and self-contained, originated at the 1904 world's fair, in St. Louis.

According to the Evanston Public Library in Illinois, the sundae was invented in Evanston around 1890 by a local druggist who added syrup on top of an ice cream soda. The city fathers felt it was so good that it was sinful to serve it on Sunday, after church. The druggist got around the ordinance by serving ice cream with syrup but without the soda. The sodaless ice cream soda was named a "sundae" to avoid confusion with "Sunday." More ice cream is sold on Sundays than on any other day of the week. A name can be a powerful thing, but the experience of ice cream can be mimicked by freezing nutritious protein-containing meal replacements. The possibilities of making healthy ice creams and even ice cream sundaes with fat-free chocolate syrup would be achievable if only there was some incentive.

What's the Point?

I could go on and on, but the point is, peanut butter, ice cream sundaes, hot dogs, burgers and fries, potato chips, and pizza are not foods that evolved slowly. Instead, they burst on the scene with all the economic energy of hula hoops, but with much more staying power. You have learned to love these tastes, but tastes can change. You can learn to appreciate healthy versions of these foods if you care about your health.

The difference between the diet encountered by humans at the time our genes developed and current times contributes significantly to obesity and many of the common chronic diseases that are epidemic today in the developed countries of the world.

The Hunter-Gatherer
Dietary Guidelines Committee

In some respects, the diet we have is pretty good. The American economy is successfully feeding a population of over 250 million, and with few exceptions, most Americans are not going to sleep hungry at night. We don't have people dying of scurvy due to a vitamin C deficiency or suffering from rickets due to a vitamin D deficiency. On the other hand, the current epidemics of diseases that arise from overnutrition and mismatches between genes and diet indicate that our diets could be a lot better.

Where historical records are available, scientists have carried out research on the eating habits and the composition of the diets of over two hundred hunter-gatherer societies. They have found that there was no single hunter-gatherer diet approved by the hunter-gatherer dietary guidelines committee. Instead, humans did their best to survive in different environments by gathering what plant foods they could and by hunting. In warmer climates there were more abundant plant foods, while in colder climates humans depended more on animal meat. At that time meat was lower in total fat and contained healthier types of fat than the grain-fed meat we eat today. In the leanest times hunter-gatherers become scavengers, eating whatever was available.

By the time our species left Africa, our genes already contained the machinery necessary to adapt to different diets. This flexibility has allowed humans to survive on extremely diverse combinations of foods. How else could it be that one population can live almost entirely on plants, while another survives mostly on whale blubber? It is reasonable to assume that such dietary diversity had some influence on the genome, as humans lived in very different surroundings around the world.

Ancient Agriculture versus
Modern Food Production and Marketing

In modern times the most significant factor in creating the rift between our genes and our diet has been the incredible success of agriculture, food processing, and food marketing. The United States 1987–1988 National Food Consumption Survey broke down the total energy (calorie) intake of all Americans as follows:

> Cereal grains: 31%
> Dairy products: 14%
> Beverages: 8%
> Oils and dressings: 4%
> Added sugar and candies: 4%

None of these foods, which together account for more than 60 percent of food intake today in the United States, was available to ancient

RELATIVE CONTRIBUTION OF PLANT FOOD TYPE TO THE WILD-PLANT FOOD DIET

TYPE OF PLANT FOOD	NUMBER*	% OF TOTAL†	ENERGY PER GRAM‡
Fruits	317	41.3	3.97
Tubers	86	11.2	4.06
Other Seeds	74	9.6	12.38
Nuts	74	9.6	12.80
Roots	51	8.5	3.93
Acacia Seeds	55	7.2	14.73
Bulbs	30	3.9	6.78
Leaves	28	3.6	2.55
Flowers	16	2.1	3.56
Miscellaneous	14	1.8	3.81
Dried Fruits	7	0.9	12.18
Gums	2	0.3	9.96

* Number: the different varieties in this category (e.g., fruits).

† % of total: the number of varieties from this category as a percentage of 768 different varieties.

‡ Energy per Gram is in kilojoules, which are the metric equivalent of calories.

humans. They are the products of agriculture, food processing, and a selection system no longer based on biology but on the economics of taste, cost, and convenience.

A survey of the diets of Australian aborigines revealed more than eight hundred different wild-plant foods. The distribution of these foods from different types of edible plants gives some idea of the diversity of plant foods in hunter-gatherer diets, as shown in the table above.

Even if we count breakfast-cereal brands as separate foods, there are few of us checking out of the supermarket with more than eight hundred different kinds of natural food. Remember, too, that a temperate, sub-tropical, or tropical rain forest or grassland had an even greater diversity of wild-plant foods than the land occupied by the Australian aborigines.

When plants grow in natural settings, they have to compete with insects, humans, other plants, and the environment to grow. The plants develop genetic defenses that include the production of chemicals that may be either beneficial or toxic to humans. But when farmers choose which plants to grow, new, more uniform species of plants are created.

This lack of genetic variation introduced by agriculture makes specific crops more susceptible to being decimated by a single pest. In the mid-1800s the Irish potato crop was destroyed by a pest, causing famine and a million deaths. In 1970, 15 percent of the U.S. corn crop was destroyed by a blight that swept through the corn belt.

The science and business of agriculture has evolved to incorporate modern industrial technologies such as automated harvesting, which works better in large, uniform fields where the plants all look alike. Agricultural science has also continued to seek out plants that grow faster, resist pests, and yield more per acre. The majority of American growers today employ powerful chemical fertilizers along with toxic pesticides and herbicides to protect crops that have not developed their own natural defenses.

It doesn't have to be this way for modern farmers. On the outskirts of Fresno, California, lie the grape fields of a sixty-three-year-old grower named Gary Pitts. His fields are easy to spot because the rows of grapevines in his fields alternate with cover crops, rows of barley, oats, and snow peas. These cover crops provide the perfect home for friendly insects that dine on grape-devouring pests. He uses almost no herbicide chemicals, but plows his cover crops into the soil so that the nitrogen in them will act as a natural fertilizer. He uses three kinds of compost in the soil, providing the plants with such good nutrition that they are able to fight off most diseases by themselves. Only as a last resort will he use chemicals—to fight off one particular pest that eats the roots of his grapevines. The soil near his plants is alive with earthworms, and his yields per acre are double those of his competitors, who spray, weed, and clean until there is no life in the soil.

Pitts operates much like the Old World farmers did. They relied on their knowledge of the land, along with some chicken manure, when growing crops. Today's agribusiness farm is tightly linked to the use of chemicals, because today's growing methods produce crops with poor defense mechanisms against disease. The use of pesticides overall has grown despite an increasingly strong organic foods movement. Some fruit tree growers in California have managed to markedly decrease their use of chemicals in the last decade, but as a world problem the use of chemicals including pesticides, herbicides, and fungicides remains an important issue.

The Culinary Melting Pot

A long series of cultural and historic events combined to give us the diet we eat today. Convenience foods have become our staples, and these foods developed out of a still-evolving multinational melting pot of cuisines. I'm not sure how our old friend *Homo erectus* would have liked Thai chicken pizza or chicken Caesar burritos, but chances are good that if he were to grow accustomed to the strong tastes and convenience of these foods, he wouldn't go back to hunting and gathering as long as these foods were available.

The process of food evolution, unlike the process of human evolution, moves rapidly and has very special characteristics. Quick advances in food evolution occur when two or more cultures meet and exchange food customs.

This type of exchange took place when herbs were first cultivated in the ancient Middle East. The mummified remains of tall Caucasian men have been found along the silk road to China, where it crosses the Gobi Desert. These men died more than three thousand years ago, when the pharaohs still ruled Egypt. They were carrying samples of a variety of spices and herbs that, many centuries later, Marco Polo would take back to Europe after his sojourns in China.

Modern Mexican cuisine comes from the mixing of the Spanish and Aztec food cultures. In the Philippines, where an Asian population had already developed a cuisine similar to that in Indonesia, the dominance of the Spanish culture influenced Filipino cuisine to a much lesser extent. To this day Filipino cuisine involves less use of chili peppers than does Mexican cuisine. In Europe the impact of tomatoes and peppers on the cuisines of Italy, Germany, France, and Hungary virtually defined national cuisines that did not exist before A.D. 1500

The American diet is also a product of history and cultural evolution. Until the Indians taught them to fertilize cornfields with fish and to raise and eat turkey, the pilgrims were close to starvation. Once the "amber waves of grain" overtook farms in the Midwest, Americans could rest assured that there would always be enough to go around. Today, cereal grains—such as wheat, corn, and rice—are a mainstay of the American diet, and have led to the widespread popularity of breakfast cereal. Those colorful boxes along the breakfast cereal aisle in the market occupy the highest-valued grocery-display space per foot of any processed food.

Many flavors and tastes that have been incorporated into the American processed-food industry were brought here by immigrant populations. Pizza, Chinese-American foods, Tex-Mex cuisine, hamburgers, hot dogs, and French fries have all been adopted, adapted, and incorporated into Americana.

Restoring Variety to Our Diets

Sure, processed foods are fun and taste great, and you can't beat them for convenience. You can purchase for under five dollars a day's worth of calories in fast food, and eat your meal while driving from one place to another. Cleaning up the mess is as easy as wadding up the wrappers and tossing them in the trash. Compared to the painstaking, time-consuming harvesting and preparation of foods our ancestors went through to survive, we have quite an easy time getting our daily nourishment.

Thirty years ago when I was a medical student, I was taught that you would get everything you needed from the four basic food groups. I was also taught that dairy products constituted the only good source of calcium, and that without red meat you were bound to be deficient in iron. According to the nutritional wisdom of that time, air-filled white bread would build my body and muscles "twelve ways" because it was enriched with twelve added vitamins and nutrients. National organizations of nutritional experts maintained that there was no such thing as "junk food," because all foods have something to offer. The world of nutrition had just begun to become an industry, and store shelves were filling with packaged and processed foods that were supposed to be every bit as good for us as food the way nature created it. Selling these packaged foods was far more profitable than doing things the old-fashioned way.

The 1950s Pleasantville Diet
Creates Diet-Book Best-Sellers

The typical diet of the fifties—high in fat and calories—didn't make sense to lots of Americans, and so a vibrant counterculture arose that embraced a different way of eating and living. These were the people who wrote and read books such as *Diet for a Small Planet* by Frances Moore Lappé, *Everything You Ever Wanted to Know About Nutrition*

But Were Afraid to Ask by David Rubin, Earl Mindell's *The Vitamin Bible*, Nathan Pritikin's *The Pritikin Diet Revolution*, and Marilyn and Harvey Diamond's *The Fit for Life Diet*.

Vitamin Supplements and Weight-Loss Industries Thrive

Nutritional supplements have become increasingly popular over the years. At one time only those on the absolute fringe used vitamins, and today more Americans use some kind of vitamin supplement than ever before. Today, 50 percent of Americans take vitamins and mineral supplements, but only 35 percent remember to take them regularly.

Weight loss continues to be an obsession, leading to an endless run of diet books that attempt to explain some secret about carbohydrates or protein as the single key to weight loss. Eating plans like the Atkins diet tell people what they want to hear. They can eat the foods they love and still lose weight. This is true, but the wide variety of phytochemicals found in fruits and vegetables is missing from the high-protein/high-fat, meat- and cheese-rich Atkins diet. If you visit your local health food store or Dr. Atkins's offices in New York, you will see that he is selling supplements to make up for the deficiencies in his diet plan. Of course, supplements don't make up for missing foods, so this diet—while it produces temporary weight loss—does not do so in a healthy way. Of course, the meat industry and the USDA are in love with this diet. It is the first diet book to have caused an increase in red-meat sales, which were slumping. Over the past five years, steak houses have been the fastest-growing restaurant category. Perhaps the photograph in *Time* magazine of Dr. Atkins slicing a big hunk of roast beef on his sixty-ninth birthday helped to convey the message that Americans who want to lose weight can now eat meat. Unfortunately for the five-foot-tall woman burning 1,200 calories per day, she gets her whole day's quota of calories in one piece of prime rib, which also has 50 grams of saturated fat.

We are indeed eating a diet that doubtless contributes to the burden of chronic disease and premature aging in our population. In order to hold on to the progress that has been made against communicable diseases, famine, and malnutrition while maintaining a truly healthy diet, we need to follow the cues of our ancestors by restoring variety to our diets. Eating a wide variety of the right types of foods is the missing piece of the puzzle that is today's nutrition controversy.

Academia and the Food Industry versus Government

Since the first dietary advice for Americans was pronounced by the government in 1915, the academic community, the food industry, and the government have been working together to provide us with the optimal diet. When we scan the colorful boxes, cans, and bottles that line supermarket shelves, we're seeing the results of this dynamic interaction among academia, the government, and food producers. As it is with any cooperative effort, however, each of these groups has its own agenda.

The academic community would like to optimize the health value of the diet through scientific advances in our understanding of human biology. Within the constraints of its survival as a profitable venture, the food industry generally operates with good intentions in this regard. Government is caught in the middle, often receiving inconsistent advice from the academic community and having to deal with the food industry's efforts to evade regulations that adversely affect its bottom line. Academia often produces more controversy than it settles in the area of nutritional science; still, on the basis of its advice, government is expected to provide guidance and regulation for the food industry and consumers.

Although it can be a difficult system to understand and participate in, its inherent checks and balances enable this trio to work together well enough to rank among the best systems of its kind in the world—but it is still not good enough. At this point in history, based on our knowledge of human genetics and nutrition, we need to adjust this system in order to update our food supply.

The Trouble with the RDA

One problem with the system is that the government tends to be extremely conservative in its nutrient recommendations, and has been slow to recognize the value of higher intakes of vitamins and minerals. Government guidelines for daily vitamin and mineral intake—the Recommended Dietary Allowances, or RDAs—have been in place for several decades.

They were never intended to suggest optimal intake, but are set above the minimum nutritional requirements needed to prevent deficiency diseases. Research on the use of vitamins and minerals in the prevention of chronic disease has consistently shown that far more than the RDA is required.

A debate that took place in the 1980s over the RDA for vitamin C is a fine example of government efforts to create dietary recommendations for Americans. The government-appointed scientists of the U.S. Food and Nutrition Board were split into two camps about recommendations for daily intake of this antioxidant vitamin. The more conservative group insisted that studies had been performed showing that only 3 percent of vitamin C is lost per day from a total body store of 1,500 milligrams. They argued that the requirement should be set at 45 milligrams per day. More progressive members of the panel felt that the intake of vitamin C from foods was too low, and that the vitamin C recommendation should be increased to 60 milligrams per day to encourage people to eat more fruit. This type of argument makes no sense when you understand that a typical orange contains 74 milligrams of vitamin C!

Dozens of reputable studies have been performed showing that much higher vitamin C intakes are quite useful in protecting the body against free radicals, and against heart disease, cancer, and infectious diseases. There is also no problem with vitamin C intakes of up to 500 milligrams per day in the vast majority of humans. The body activates genes that cause any extra vitamin C to be excreted in the urine.

The Politics of Nutrition

When business, science, and government interact to provide the public with dietary recommendations, the facts can quickly become buried beneath slick advertising and the efforts of corporate lobbyists. The ups and downs of the dairy industry are a good example. At one time the government provided subsidies, which have since expired, to the dairy industry to encourage milk production. At the time they were introduced, there was a great push to communicate the health benefits of milk, particularly with regards to its central role in providing calcium for healthy bones. The government aided the dairy industry in these promotions, advising Americans to eat dairy products for the calcium they contain. The dairy industry soon learned that health messages don't sell milk, and haven't had any better luck with the "white mustache" and

"Got milk?" campaigns that followed. At the same time, the fruit juice industry—again, with government support—has supplemented orange juice and tomato juice with calcium in its citrate/malate form, which academia has found to be more available to the body than the calcium found in milk.

If you recall the earlier discussion of how ancient humans made their food choices, you'll see how far into consumer culture we've strayed from our slowly evolving genetic programming. Our food choices are no longer related to our genetics or to biology, but are imposed by government, academia, and industry. As these parties collaborate to establish dietary guidelines, advertisers shape cultural evolution, using the tactics of applied psychology to persuade consumers that certain products will enrich their lives, their relationships, and their health.

Choosing New Foods Is Still Possible

The variety and diversity of the diet moves much more quickly than any genome can optimally accommodate. Still, it is possible to integrate new scientific information about our food supply and our genetics as it emerges. This is already happening, as the business of marketing foods to the public is shaped by the needs and desires of consumers.

When consumers told the food industry that they did not like brown spots on their French fries, a potato was bred that would yield perfect, golden fries without any brown spots. Today, all of the French fries in the United States are made from russet Burbank potatoes. A perfect French fry is made in a programmed cooker by immersing it in very hot oil. Originally, this oil included lard as a secret ingredient. After that, hydrogenated soybean oil was produced to provide the same heat stability at high temperatures. Now French fry makers could advertise that the French fries were cholesterol-free and made with 100 percent vegetable oil, thus having been adapted to current consumer demands.

The Story of Olestra, the Fat-Free Fat

In the 1980s low-fat diets came into vogue, and the food industry exploded with over one thousand different fat-free foods as consumer demand for them rose. To make these foods as tasty as their full-fat counterparts, food manufacturers simply replaced the calories from fat with added sugar. The appeal of sweetness to the human taste buds helped the low-fat, high-sugar sales boom. Some foods, such as Snack-well cookies, found themselves struggling to compete with the "real" cookies while trying to become as fat-free and calorie-free as possible. At the end of the 1980s, the "fat free" fat, Olestra, finally came on the market, but was restricted by the FDA to the so-called savory snack-food category of chips. This food engineering marvel behaved like fat but was not absorbed into the body. Made up of fatty acids attached to the six corners of a sucrose molecule, this fat is resistant to the digestive process that usually splits the fatty acids off the three-carbon triglyceride molecule in ordinary dietary fats and oils.

While this invention had some promise, it was kept at bay for years by a combination of cooking-oil interests until it finally received its restricted approval. Then the rumor was floated that it caused diarrhea; a controlled study using popcorn made with the usual oils or Olestra showed that this was simply not true. Unfortunately, it was too late. While no one was getting sick from these chips made with Olestra, the low-fat era was over and the era of Dr. Atkins had begun.

Agriculture Responds to Consumers

Recently, when consumers were told by scientists at Harvard that trans-fatty acids from hydrogenated oils could threaten their health, the government dictated that all foods containing these oils should have their trans-fat content indicated on the label. Farmers then responded by developing a new strain of soybean that yields oil with a lower linoleic-acid content, can be used without hydrogenation, and lasts longer on the shelf.

The consumer has demanded fruits and vegetables that don't look spoiled or rotten. That means harvesting fruits and vegetables while they are still firm and unblemished. While these plant foods are able to withstand the long trip to market, they often have reduced taste and reduced levels of health-giving phytochemicals. For example, hothouse tomatoes have more lycopene (the red pigment) than the usual ethylene-sprayed green tomato you buy in the store.

The Consumer Is King

When consumers communicate what they want, the industry and government will, ultimately, respond. In each of the cases mentioned above, the industry did its best to produce good-tasting foods that would sell. Some attempt was made to incorporate current knowledge about the relationship between food and health, but in most instances this tended to be a secondary concern.

Modern industrial society has significantly narrowed our typical food choices, and our busy lifestyles have done the rest. We have cheated our genes of the chance to evolve to where they can interact with this new diet. Consumers too often decide what they want based on habit, convenience, and the strong, even addictive tastes and textures of foods that have had most of their nutritional value processed out and unhealthful ingredients added in.

A shift is occurring, however, as more and more people make food choices based on reliable information about what is best for them. As consumers move in this direction, the food industry will have no choice but to create products that fulfill our needs.

The Prevention Prescription
Is Optimizing Our Diets

Now that rickets, scurvy, pellagra, and other deficiency diseases have been conquered, and now that increased food availability has helped stem the tide of infectious diseases that flourish in malnourished populations, nature has placed a new hurdle in the path of humanity: the chronic diseases of aging. If you are out in the bush worrying about where your next meal is coming from, the diseases of aging are not on your mind. But it's unlikely that you are starving or severely vitamin deficient in this day and age, so we now have the opportunity as never before in human history to turn our attention to finding out how to live a longer, healthier life.

The prevention of chronic disease by adding diverse fruits and vegetables to the diet requires a whole new view of dietary guidelines. Dietary guidelines such as the RDA have traditionally been designed to provide adequate nutrition to avoid deficiency diseases, but they were never designed to recommend diets for optimal health. To simplify the labeling of foods so that separate RDAs would not have to be listed for men and women at different ages, a composite USRDA was developed, with a single set of calorie and nutrient recommendations. I like to joke that this was designed for a thirty-year-old pregnant male! The diversity of the human genome is such that guidelines based on gender and age groups of typical individuals will no longer suffice. The foods we eat interact intimately with our genes, and can increase or decrease our risk of chronic disease.

As you learn more about the miracles of medicine just over the horizon, remember the principles and lessons of this book. The promises of the new era of biotechnology can be fulfilled only if we commit our society to a new era of health-education that promotes more self-care, and only if we take the responsibility for reinventing agriculture to provide foods and herbs for health.

Appendix 1: Determining Your Calorie and Protein Requirement

Your genes determine, to a large extent, your requirement for dietary protein. One of the most important genetic determinants is whether you are male or female. For weight and height women almost always have more fat and less lean body mass—tissues that are not stored fat—than do men. Maintenance of muscle tissue requires more calories and more protein than maintenance of fat, and so women require fewer calories and less protein to stay at the same weight. The formula I'm going to give you to calculate your own calorie and protein intake will take this and other genetic differences into account.

For over fifteen years I have been using an instrument called a "bioelectrical impedance analyzer" in my nutritional-medicine clinic. With this instrument I can measure lean body mass and estimate daily calorie requirements. The test is simple and requires only that the patient take off shoes and socks. Gel electrodes, exactly like those used for taking electrocardiograms, are placed on the hands and feet, and a very mild electrical current is sent into the body. Muscle is about 70 percent water and conducts electricity; fat is an insulator and does not conduct electricity. The differences in conduction between the two types of tissue provide the machine with a measurement of electrical impedance, which it plugs into a formula that calculates lean body mass. Once we know the lean body mass, it is simple to calculate fat mass and percentage body fat.

You will be using another equation to calculate your calorie needs, based on the amount of lean body mass you're carrying. It's as simple as multiplying the number of pounds of lean body mass by fourteen to arrive at the number of calories burned per day at rest. This is your resting metabolic rate.

A woman with a lean body mass of 100 pounds will expend 1,400 calories a day at rest. Let's say her husband is carrying 150 pounds of lean tissue; he'll burn up 2,100 calories a day at rest. Now it so happens that in this example, the woman is 5 feet 2 inches tall, while her husband is 5 feet 10 inches tall. Men who are taller than women will usually have more lean body mass. If they sit down together to a hearty meal of prime rib, vegetables, salad, and dessert—amounting to 1,300 to 1,500 calories—the husband will get a good portion of his daily requirement, but his wife will have gone into caloric surplus for the day. On the other hand, I have seen some women with more lean mass than men. I have one woman patient who is 5 feet 10 inches tall and weighs 300 pounds but has a lean body mass of 180 pounds. She has a resting metabolic rate of 2,520 calories per day. She will have an easier time losing weight on the same diet as either the husband or wife in the above example.

Both men and women naturally experience changes in muscle and fat distribution as they age, and calorie needs decrease accordingly. Muscle mass decreases and fat mass increases, often despite all efforts to prevent this shift. By the fourth decade of life, all but the most conscientious (or genetically gifted) can expect to experience some form of "middle-aged spread." This is especially true as physical activity levels decline and bad eating habits continue as a matter of course.

As you can probably guess by now, my prescription for protein will not be an exact one. I can't tell you to eat three strawberries, a raspberry, and a banana to meet your vitamin requirements, and I also can't tell you the exact amount of protein to eat. If your estimate is in the ballpark, you will be eating enough protein to satiate your appetite and to balance the pancreatic insulin response to carbohydrates. You'll also have enough protein coming in to maintain your muscle mass (with regular exercise).

Knowing your lean body mass is the first step in estimating your basal metabolic rate, the number of pounds you will lose if you diet, and the target weight you should aim for. The most practical way to measure your lean mass is with the bioelectrical impedance analyzer I mentioned above. Call around to local gyms, fitness centers, and doctors' offices, and set up an appointment to have the measurement done. In specialty gadget stores you can find body-fat meters with metal plates that you stand on with bare feet or hold with your hands. These aren't quite as accurate as the instrument I use in my office, but they will still give you a good estimate of your lean mass.

Once you have had this measurement done, you can plug the number into this formula:

Lean body mass $\times$ 14 calories/day = resting metabolic rate (RMR)

The RMR represents how many calories you burn at rest per day. Once you know this number, you're within 25 percent of the total calories you should consume per day. Now consider whether you have struggled to control your weight in the past. If you have, take the RMR as your total calorie needs. Adding daily exercise to your life, if you haven't already, will boost your calorie expenditure above your intake, and you'll lose weight. If you are thin and athletic, multiply the RMR by 1.25 to estimate your calorie needs.

Now you can move on to estimating your protein requirement. Most people do well with one gram of protein per pound of lean body mass per day.

Lean body mass $\times$ 1 = grams protein needed per day

All proteins, however, are not created equal. The proteins you eat are made up of various combinations of twenty-one amino acids. Of those twenty-one, nine are essential—humans need to consume them in foods to stay free of amino-acid-deficiency diseases. The nonessential amino acids can be made in the body from the essential ones.

Protein foods are ranked on a 100-point scale. The ideal mixture of amino acids for human protein needs is found in egg whites, and this food earns a score of 100. It contains all of the essential amino acids, and is easily digested and processed in the body. Casein, a protein from milk, is nearly as good, with a score of 99. Soy protein has almost as good an amino-acid profile as animal foods, and earns a high score of nearly 100. Red meat, chicken, and fish are scored at 80, while corn and beans each score only 20 to 40 when eaten alone. If corn and beans are combined, their collective score goes up to 80 because their amino acids complement one another.

Proteins from plants lack enough of certain amino acids to meet our genetic requirements. The remains of groups of purely vegetarian prehuman primates have shown us that they could not compete with our omnivorous, hunter-gatherer ancestors. In light of our genetic similarities to other animal species, it makes sense that animal proteins would better meet our protein requirements. Plant proteins can be combined to complement one another's incomplete essential amino-acid content, providing a so-called complete protein. You can do this by combining grains or seeds with beans. Try black beans and rice, lentil or split pea soup and whole-grain bread, corn tortillas and pinto beans, or hummus (garbanzo beans mixed with sesame seed paste).

Appendix 2: Tools

For those who are on the Web, this is a website you can use to enhance your reading of this book.

- www.Miavita.com: I am a scientific adviser to this site, which provides recipes and tools to complement the approach in this book for losing weight and enhancing your diet through the Color Code.

There are also tools you can use to enhance your appreciation of this book:

- Bioelectrical Impedance Analysis: This can be done by physicians who have quadripolar machines. Some manufacturers of these accurate machines, which are different from what is found in department stores, are RJL, Inc. in Detroit, Michigan, and Biodynamics, Inc. in Seattle, Washington. There are no standards set by the government for approving these machines, but these are widely used and have been validated in some of our research studies. Information obtained from one of these machines is critical in using the preceding Appendix 1.
- Pedometers: These can be obtained at any electrical novelty store and some department stores. They have digital electronic counters and sense the movement of an internal device that registers whenever you step. The accuracy is high, but the amount of energy burned varies from one person to another. So set a personal goal and meet it each day.

Recommended Reading
and References

The references I used for writing this book were many. It would be inappropriate to reference every sentence as if this were one of my scientific papers. However, I wanted to give the reader the opportunity to research further topics of interest that naturally followed from this text. For those readers who want to chase down some of the original references, I have annotated most of the references to indicate the information that was drawn from a particular source.

INTRODUCTION

Harper, Alfred E. (ed.). "Physiologically Active Food Components." *American Journal of Clinical Nutrition* (supplement) no. 6S (June 2000): 1,647S–1,743S.

This journal supplement is available from the American Society for Clinical Nutrition, Inc., in Rockville, Maryland, and represents the report of the 17th Ross Research Conference on Medical Issues held in San Diego, California, from February 22 to 24, 1998. An excellent article by Dr. John Milner on functional foods, from the U.S. perspective, influenced my thinking in developing the Color Code and the concepts expressed in the introduction.

1. WHAT COLOR IS YOUR DIET?

Broekmans, W.M.R.; I.A.A. Ketelaars Klopping; C.R.W.C. Schuurman; H. Verhagen; H. Van den Berg; F. J. Kok; and G. van Poppel. "Fruits and vegetables increase plasma carotenoids and vitamins and decrease homocysteine in humans." *Journal of Nutrition* 130 (2000): 1578–1583.

This study demonstrated the effects of increasing fruit and vegetable intake from 100 grams per day to 500 grams per day. Combined with my knowledge of the cancer-prevention literature, this article brought home to me the practicality of recommending a variety of fruits and vegetables to improve health. The ability of these researchers to reach the 500 gram goal with diets that appeared practical greatly impressed me.

2. COLORIZING YOUR DIET

Sears, Barry. *A Week in the Zone*. New York: ReganBooks, 2000.

While working on my book, I picked up this paperback at an airport gift shop and was stunned at how clearly it was written for the lay public. The advice was clear and concise, and unlike most scientific papers I read and write. I decided to use the organization of the practical advice in this book to frame my discussion for the practical steps to starting this diet, shopping for foods, traveling, and dining in restaurants. I added my own advice and used some of the general advice this book adapted from common wisdom. Incidentally, I don't disagree with what is written in the *Zone* diet. What made this book so popular was the realization that certain high-fat foods could be eaten and still be consistent with losing weight. The book was attacked as a high-protein book, but it was really written to make the distinction between high-fiber carbohydrates and refined carbohydrates. My book takes this many steps further by basing the diet on fruits and vegetables instead of cereals and grains. I also provide a variety of different groups of fruits and vegetables to take advantage of the different physiological mechanisms by which fruits and vegetables can work. Incidentally, I was also aware of the dangers of oversimplification of complex concepts. Barry Sears's entire zone concept applies to a subset of individuals who are prediabetic and doesn't apply to the majority of Americans. Insulin does play an important role, but as I point out, it is not the whole story.

3. USING THE COLOR CODE

Heber, David. *The Resolution Diet*. New York: Avery Books, 1999.

I used many of the ideas in my previous book to help people implement a low-fat diet based on portion control. I have used my experience in clinical medicine and nutrition in both books. The ideas I am using are the ones I teach to physicians and use with patients myself at UCLA.

4. TRAVELING AND DINING WITH THE COLOR CODE

Brownell, K. D., and T. A. Wadden. *The LEARN Program for Weight Control*. Dallas, Tex.: American Health Publishing Company, 1998.

Covey, S. R. *First Things First*. New York: Fireside, 1994.

In this chapter I used a combination of my own ideas from *The Resolution Diet* and some of the behavioral principles and practical techniques in the above two books. Many of the ideas are drawn from advice appearing in The LEARN Program developed by Dr. Kelly Brownell and Dr. Tom Wadden. The set of twenty-four lessons includes ways to gradually introduce new habits, tolerate your predictable lapses, and work toward a new way of life. I also incorporated the philosophies inherent in Steven Covey's book *Seven Habits of Highly Effective People* in all its variations. His book *First Things First* is a practical guide on getting his system going, which I highly recommend.

5. GETTING OFF THE COUCH

American Heart Association. *Fitting in Fitness*. New York: Times Books, 1997.

For sheer numbers of suggestions, this small paperback takes the cake. There are numerous charts and workbook examples to urge you to get off the couch and get active. Combining this book with a pedometer is the best thing you can do to increase your energy burning. Once you have mastered walking, the next step is bodybuilding. The information in this chapter was taken from my own experience since 1977 of weight lifting. I was more successful and rigorous when I was younger, but I was not as busy then. In fact, I experienced the exhilaration in the 1970s of building muscle, which I hope you will experience.

6. SUPPLEMENTS: PILLS AND FOODS FOR HEALTH

Chandra, R. K. "Effect of vitamin and trace-element supplementation on immune response and infections in elderly subjects." *Lancet* 340 (1992): 1,124–1,127.

"Homocysteine Lowering Trialists' Collaboration: Lowering blood homocysteine with folic acid–based supplements: meta-analysis of randomized trials." *British Medical Journal* 316 (1998): 894–898.

Institute of Medicine, Food and Nutrition Board. *Dietary Reference Intakes for Thiamin, Riboflavin, Niacin, Vitamin B_6, Folate, Vitamin B_{12}, Pantothenic Acid, Biotin, and Choline*. Washington, D.C.: National Academy Press, 1998.

Meydani S. N.; M. Meydani; and J. B. Blumber, et al. "Vitamin E supplementation and in vivo immune response in healthy elderly subjects: a randomized controlled trial." *Journal of the American Medical Association* 277 (1997): 1,380–1,386.

Packer, L.; M. Hiramatsu; and T. Yoshikawa. *Antioxidant Food Supplements in Human Health*. San Diego, Calif.: Academic Press, 1999.

Weaver, C.; W. R., Proulx; and R. Heaney. "Choices for achieving adequate dietary calcium with a vegetarian diet." *American Journal of Clinical Nutrition* 70 (1999): 543s-548s.

The book by Packer, Hiramatsu, and Yoshikawa is an excellent collection of scientific chapters on antioxidants in connection with disease, including information on alpha-lipoic acid you will not find elsewhere. The paper by Weaver, et al. contains tables demonstrating the bioavailability of calcium from fortified orange juice, tofu, and vegetables. The other papers listed are some of the many references on the new ways to use of vitamin and mineral supplements that enhance immune function and reduce the risk of disease.

7. DISCOVERING THE WORLD OF PLANT FOODS

DeWitt, D., and B. W. Bosland. *The Pepper Garden.* New York: Ten Speed Press, 1993.

DeBaggio, T. *Growing Herbs.* Loveland, Colo.: Interweave Press, 1994.

Kowalchik, C., ed. *Rodale's Illustrated Encyclopedia of Herbs.* Emmaus, Pa.: Rodale Press, 1987.

Norman, J. *The Complete Book of Spices.* New York: Viking Studio Books, 1991.

If you liked what you read in this chapter, you have a lot more exploring to do. I was not able to include all the wonderful fruits and vegetables that you should discover. So pick up one of these guides and continue the adventure.

8. THE FIFTEEN MOST COMMON MYTHS ABOUT NUTRITION

Heber, David. *The Resolution Diet.* New York: Avery Books, 1999.

Yetiv, Jack Z. *Popular Nutritional Practices: A Scientific Appraisal.* Toledo, Ohio: Popular Medicine Press, 1986.

Most of the myths were discussed in my earlier book on dieting, especially the various diet myths. The information on food mislabeling and misinformation is my own observation, gleaned over the last twenty years in the field, and has been supplemented by a number of analyses based on scientific principles and outlined in the book by Jack Yetiv, M.D., Ph.D. written fifteen years ago.

9. HOW DNA DAMAGE LEADS TO DISEASE

Bland, J. S. *Genetic Nutritioneering.* Los Angeles, Calif.: Keats Publishing, 1999.

This well-written book lays out the arguments for our nutrition having an impact on genetic expression and the ultimate occurrence of common diseases. A detailed account of the discovery of homocysteine by Kilmer McCully leads to a discussion of the impact of nutrition on genetic susceptibility to heart disease.

10. THE SURPRISING FAT CELL: MUCH MORE THAN A BAG OF FAT

Gao, Y.; Q. Yang; and J. Zhou. "Association between leptin, insulin, and body fat distribution in type 2-diabetes mellitus." *Annals of the New York Academy of Sciences* 904 (May 2000): 542–545.

Kirkland, J. L.; C. H. Hollenberg; and W. S. Gillon. "Effects of fat depot site on differentiation-dependent gene expression in rat preadipocytes." *International Journal of Obesity and Related Metabolic Disorders,* supplement 3 (March 1996): S102–S107.

Matsuzawa, Y.; T. Funahashi; and T. Nakamura. "Molecular mechanism of metabolic syndrome X: contribution of adipocytokines, adipocyte-derived bioactive substances." *Annals of the New York Academy of Sciences* 892 (November 18, 1999): 146–154.

These three review articles describe some of the functions of the surprising fat cell, which I describe. There are other papers in this area, but this small collection will be a good start. This subject is not treated in a textbook, because the information is still too new.

11. HEART DISEASE, CHOLESTEROL, AND YOUR DNA

Heber, D. *Natural Remedies for a Healthy Heart*. New York: Avery Publishing Group, 1998.

Kullo, I. J.; G. T. Gau; and A. J. Takik. "Novel Risk Factors for Atherosclerosis." *Mayo Clinic Proceedings* 75 (2000): 369–380.

Lefer, D. J., and N. Granger. "Oxidative Stress and Cardiac Disease." *American Journal of Medicine* 109 (2000): 315–323.

My first book, *Natural Remedies for a Healthy Heart*, details a modern view of heart disease and how it progresses. It also discusses a number of natural remedies, including Chinese red yeast rice. The review article by Lefer and Granger is an up-to-date view of oxidation and heart disease that includes information on nitric oxide and inflammation, and the review by Kullo, Gau, and Tajik at the Mayo Clinic outlines the evidence for recognized novel risk factors for heart disease, including homocysteine; fibrinogen; lipoprotein(a); small, dense LDL; and inflammatory-infectious markers.

12: CANCER IS A DNA DISEASE

Heber, D.; G. L. Blackburn; and V.L.W. Go. *Nutritional Oncology*. San Diego, Calif.: Academic Press, 1999.

Lee, W. H.; W. B. Isaacs; G. S. Bova; and W. G. C. G. Nelson. "Island Methylation Changes Near the GSTP1 Gene in Prostatic Carcinoma Cells Detected Using the Polymerase Chain Reaction: A New Prostatic Cancer Biomarker." *Cancer Epidemiology, Biomarkers and Prevention* 6 (1997): 443–450.

The textbook on nutritional oncology, which I edited with Dr. Blackburn and Dr. Go, is a comprehensive text that demonstrates the many aspects of the gene-nutrient interaction in cancer and the role of oxidative stress in this disease. The paper by Lee et al., from Johns Hopkins University, demonstrates the genetic damage to the antioxidant system in prostate cancer cells, which is key to understanding gene-nutrient interaction.

13. AGING, SEX DRIVE, MENTAL FUNCTION, AND YOUR DNA

Ly, D. H.; D. J. Lockhart; R. A. Lerner; and P. G. Schultz. "Mitotic misregulation and human aging." *Science* 287 (2000): 2,486–2,492.

In this study cells from children with premature aging were compared to cells from normal youngsters and cells from elderly individuals. The mutations found on oxidative-protection genes and quality-control or checkpoint genes give an insight into the process of aging.

14. GENE-DIET IMBALANCE AND DAMAGE TO DNA

Diamond, Jared. *The Third Chimpanzee*. New York: HarperPerennial, 1992.

Owens, K., and M. C. King. "Genomic Views of Human History." *Science* 286 (1999): 451–453.

The review article by Mary-Claire King and Kelly Owens is part of the genome issue of *Science* magazine that changed my thinking about human evolution. I discovered *The Third Chimpanzee* by Jared Diamond, professor of physiology at UCLA, and learned a great deal that influenced my writings in this area.

15. CULTURAL EVOLUTION AND THE LOSS OF EDEN

Diamond, Jared. *Guns, Germs, and Steel.* New York: W. W. Norton and Company, 1999.

Eaton, S. B., and M. Konner. "Paleolithic nutrition. A consideration of its nature and current implications." *New England Journal of Medicine* 312 (1985): 283–289.

Dr. Jared Diamond is a valued colleague at UCLA and his book deservedly won the Pulitzer Prize and the *L. A. Times* Book Prize. Its treatment of cultural evolution and the impact of agriculture on human societies is described in detail. This book greatly affected my thought processes and provided much information useful in the formulation of my own ideas in this area. I highly recommend this book to anyone interested in the topics discussed in this chapter. The paper by S. B. and M. Konner Eaton describes the implications for the health of modern man based on the imbalance of our genes and our environment, information gleaned from an examination of the diets of paleolithic times.

16. FOOD EVOLUTION AND AGRICULTURAL ECONOMICS

Cordain, L.; J. B. Miller; S. B. Eaton; N. Mann; S.H.A. Holt; and J. D. Speth. "Plant-animal subsistence ratios and macronutrient energy estimations in worldwide hunter-gatherer diets." *American Journal of Clinical Nutrition* 71 (2000): 682–692.

Sims, L. S. *The Politics of Fat.* New York: M.E. Sharpe, 1998.

The book by Sims explains how government policy in the United States is formulated to affect our food supply, and it details the negotiations around the USDA pyramid by the food industry and the Department of Agriculture during the Reagan administration in the mid-1980s. This is must reading for anyone who is interested in the political aspects of changing the agricultural and food economy in the United States. The scientific paper by Cordain and coworkers documents the diversity of hunter-gatherer diets and is the source of the information in the text on this subject.

Acknowledgments

I am blessed by a convergence, in the beautiful southern California sunshine, of support from my family, my friends, my colleagues, and my patients. It is within this Mediterranean climate of creation that the ideas for this book were formed. I want to thank my wife, Anita, and my children, Marc and Adrianna, for supporting me during my hours of typing away at my computer in my home office. I want to thank Susan Bowerman, M.S., R.D., the assistant director of the UCLA Center for Human Nutrition, without whose support, contributions, and efforts this book would not have been possible. She wrote all the recipes, and served as a sounding board for me as I challenged accepted nutritional dogma on the basis of science and physiology.

I want to thank those individuals, including S. Daniel Abraham, Michael Milken, Lowell Milken, Haim Saban, Raymond Stark, Dr. Edward Steinberg, Dennis A. Tito, Dr. Scott Connelly, Henry Burdick, Andy Grove, Art Kern, and Beth Kobliner, whose contributions of resources, inspiration, and support have made the UCLA Center for Human Nutrition a reality in the short time since its founding in 1996.

No book rises from original thought without precedence, and I would like to thank those thought leaders who influenced me most in writing this book. Dr. Jared Diamond, professor of physiology at UCLA whose books *Guns, Germs, and Steel* and *The Third Chimpanzee* told the story of human evolution, and the development of agriculture and the domestication of foods, inspiring my approach to better matching our diets to our genes. Professor Stephen Jay Gould's book *Full House* laid out the nature of evolution in detailed academic terms, and provided a foundation for the validity of the arguments I have made about human evolution, cultural evolution, and diet. The description in *Science* magazine of the impact of the genomics revolution on medicine on a weekly basis has continued to energize me as I have read each new development.

While I was writing this book, I also had the responsibility for directing the activities of the UCLA Center for Human Nutrition, conducting an active research program involving two NIH-funded centers and a training grant, and organizing the annual meeting of the North American Association for the Study of Obesity. I could not have maintained these activities without the assistance of my close colleagues Drs. Vay Liang Go, Ian Yip, Zhao-Ping Li, Robert M. Elashoff, Diane Harris, Phil Koeffler, Audra Lembertas, Jake Lusis, Qing-Yi Lu, Susanne Henning, Julio Licinio, Mai Nguyen, Ma-Li Wong, and their research fellows and staff.

I also want to thank Doug Corcoran, my editor at ReganBooks, for his guidance and help in pulling this book in a direction that made it far more accessible to the general public. Originally written as an academic treatise entitled *Eat for Your Genes*, it would have spoken to a much smaller audience. I also want to thank Virginia Hopkins for her editorial and writing contributions to the earlier version of this book. My greatest appreciation goes to Judith Regan, whose belief in the message of this book and whose creative contributions have driven this process from the beginning.

Index

Page numbers in *italics* refer to illustrations.

acorns, 220–21
addictions, 206–7
age-related diseases, 172, 193–98, 244–45
  Alzheimer's disease, 8, 9, 12, 13, 103,
    138, 187, 197–98
  cataracts, 15, 18, 187, 193–94
  fractures, 191, 194, 195
  macular degeneration, xv, 15, 18, 187,
    193–94
  osteoporosis, 93, 187, 193, 194–95
  see also cancer; heart disease
aging, elderly, xiii, 8, 9, 12, 13, 97, 100,
    167, 172–73, 175, 186–98, 211
  antioxidants for, 190–91, 193–94, 197–98
  avoiding falls in, 195
  calorie restriction for, 190
  causes of, 186–87
  checkpoint genes in, 189
  gastrointestinal problems in, 191
  genetic factors in, 188–89, 192–93, 198
  increased body mass index in, 191
  life span and, 187, 188, 190, 192–93
  lowered sex drive in, 195–97
  maintaining vision and, 193–94
  memory loss in, 197–98
  premature, 138, 189, 190, 192, 239
  supplements for, 190–91, 192, 193–94, 198

  telomere shortening in, 188–89
  theories of, 187–90
agriculture, 214, 220–24, 234–36, 243
  domestication in, 221–23
  in early New England, 223–24
  hybrid corn in, 224
  in Midwest, 224
  in New World, 222, 223
  pesticide use in, 236
Albright, Fuller, 194–95
alpha-carotenes, 17, 151
alpha lipoic acid, 97, 190–91, 198
Alzheimer's disease, 8, 9, 12, 13, 103,
    138
  antioxidants and, 197–98
Ames, Bruce, 190
Amgen, 149
animal domestication, 221–22
anthocyanins, 16–17, 97
antibiotics, 98–99
antioxidants, 16–17, 18, 87, 92, 96, 97,
    120, 137, 159, 166, 169, 179, 209
  aging and, 190–91, 193–94, 197–98
  Alzheimer's disease and, 197–98
  cancer and, 176–77, 182
  in DNA defense system, 138, 139–41,
    142–43

antioxidants *(cont'd)*
    fat cell storage of, 148, 150–51
    supplemental, 92, 177, 190–91, 198
aphrodisiacs, 197
apolipoprotein B, 163–65
apoptosis, 171–72
aryl hydrocarbon receptor (AhR), 178
aspirin, 89, 144, 161, 169, 183
As You Like It (Shakespeare), 198
atherosclerosis, 9, 97, 142, 146, 160,
    165–66, 196
Atkins diet, 239, 243
atrophic gastritis, 142
Australian aborigines, 235
autoimmune diseases, 168
avocados, 15, 18, 76, 108, 144, 146, 197

babies:
    nutrition of, 201–3
    premature, 137
    small, 153, 201, 202
    spina bifida in, 93, 201
baby formula, 202–3
bacteria, 5–6, 98–99, 142, 143, 168, 191,
    216
    pro-biotic, 183–84
bananas, 107
    as fattening, 129
barbecue dinner, 25, 31
basic four food groups, 93, 95, 128–29, 220,
    238
basil, 116
bergamot, 116
beta-carotenes, 17, 94, 111, 142, 151
binge-eating disorder, 208–9
biomarkers, 182
bisque, tomato-soy, 22, 27, 47, 52
Black, Homer, 182–83
black tea, 96, 97, 180
blood-brain barrier, 197–98, 207
blood clots, 17, 160, 161, 167–68
body fat, xvi, 14, 148–56, 203, 210
    distribution of, 151–52, 155, 210, 211
    excess, 150, 155–56
    optimal percentage of, 155
    percentage of, 150
    set-point of, 210–11
    see also fat cells
body mass index, 191
bone turnover, 194
brain:
    appetite center of, 149, 153, 202, 232
    dopamine in, 206–7

endorphins in, 120, 127
    pleasure center of, 206–7, 208
    serotonin in, 207
breakfast burritos, 23, 29, 47, 60
business trips, 83, 88

cabbage:
    and bell pepper slaw, 23, 29, 47, 57–58
    sweet-and-sour stuffed, 24, 30, 47, 66–67
cafeteria diet, 149, 210
calcium, 41, 95, 128, 129, 180, 194, 201,
    225, 238, 241–42
    cheese crackers as source of, 19, 132
    deficiency of, 93
    supplemental, 19, 192
California, biodiversity of, 220–21
California Cuisine Pyramid, 121, 225–27,
    226
calories, xv, xvi, 87, 124, 127–28, 130, 169,
    211
    calculating requirement for, 13–14,
    247–49
    in fats, 121, 144
    fat storage of, 148
    in nuts, 46
    restriction of, 170, 176, 190
cancer, xiii, xvii, 3, 5, 8, 9, 11, 12, 13, 18,
    97, 125, 148, 150, 167, 171–85,
    188–89, 190, 193, 212, 241
    angiogenesis inhibitors of, 96
    antioxidants and, 176–77, 182
    biomarkers and, 182
    breast, xvi, 8, 96, 102, 145, 174, 175,
    176, 179, 184–85, 209
    calorie restriction for, 176
    carcinogens and, 140, 175, 176, 178, 181,
    184
    cervical, 185
    chemotherapy for, 182
    colon, xvi, 144, 169, 174, 179, 184, 185
    developmental stages of, 172, 173–74
    diet and, 118, 172, 173, 175, 176, 177,
    178–83
    dietary preventives of, 179–82
    as disease of civilization, 172–73
    early detection of, 173, 184–85
    esophageal, 179
    fats and, 182–83
    genetic factors in, 171–72, 173, 174, 177,
    178–79, 218
    infections in, 142
    inflammation in, 144, 168, 169, 183
    lung, 139–40, 172, 178, 179

metastasis of, 174
micronutrients and, 179–82
ovarian, 140
overeating and, 209
oxygen radicals in, 138, 139–40, 141
pro-biotic bacteria and, 183–84
prostate, xvi, 8, 96, 102, 140, 145, 174, 175, 179, 182
rates of, 172–73
risk factors for, 172, 173, 174–75, 178–80, 218
smoking and, 139–40, 172, 177–78
stomach, 140, 142, 168, 179
telomerase and, 188–89
uterine, 140, 185
vaginal, 202
canola oil, 41, 45, 146
capsaicin, 45, 119
carbohydrates, 9, 18, 20, 91–92
cravings for, 207
desirable vs. undesirable, 18–19
refined, 14, 20, 40, 45, 125–26, 225
removal of, 40
carnosic acid, 118
carotenoids, 16, 17, 18, 181
carrots, 6, 17, 45, 129, 150–51
as fattening, 129
cashews, 121
cataracts, 15, 18, 187, 193–94
catechins, 79, 96, 97
cells, 6, 158, 166
apoptosis of, 171–72
bone, 194
divisions of, 188, 189, 209
egg, 216
muscle, 86–87, 92, 97, 142
overproduction of, 13, 142
oxygen radicals in, 176–77
cereal, soy nugget, with fruit, 21, 26
chef's salad with balsamic vinaigrette, 25, 31, 47, 69
chestnuts, 120–21
chicken:
breast seven color salad, 21, 26, 47, 48–49
and brown rice bowl, 24, 29, 47, 61–62
chili peppers, 45, 119–20, 197, 223, 237
China, 101, 102, 106, 109, 110, 112, 114, 204, 214, 223, 231, 232, 237
Chinese red yeast rice, 99, 160, 163
Chinese restaurants, 78–79, 110
chives, 116
cholesterol, 108, 120, 121, 139, 141–42, 157–70, 230

apolipoprotein B and, 163–65
description of, 158–60
functions of, 158
HDL, 159, 164
in human evolution, 158–59, 161
LDL, 97, 159, 160, 163–64, 167
in plant-based diet, 158–59, 161, 162, 164
in plaque formation, 160–61, 168, 169
cholesterol, blood levels of, 102, 146, 157–58, 159–60
genetic factors in, 159, 161–64
myths about, 130–31
plant compounds for, 163
red yeast rice for, 99, 160, 163
regulation of, 162–63
cholesterol-lowering drugs, 7–8, 99, 157–58, 160, 163, 164
choline, 178
chopped vegetable salad, 22, 28, 47, 54–55
chromosomes, 5, 165, 176, 188, 189
X, 216
Y, 215–17
cod, pan-seared, with balsamic vinegar and thyme, 22, 27, 47, 53
Cohanim, 216
Color Code, xv, 5, 9–12, 13–74, 147
calorie requirement in, 13–14
choices for, 43
color groups in, 16–18, 17, 44; see also specific color groups
controlling fat intake in, 14–15
desirable vs. undesirable foods in, 18–19
diet plans in, 20–42
dinner plate redesigned in, 41–43, 42
excess body fat reduced by, 155–56
menus for, 21–32
plant food diversity in, 106–22
protein intake in, 14
recipes for, 47–69
and removal of undesirable foods, 39–41
serving as defined in, 107, 115–16
shopping list for, 70–74
staples of, 45–47
copper, 94, 120
corn, hybrid, 224
corn oil, 3, 40, 130, 144, 146, 224
couscous, whole-wheat, 22, 46
Culpeper, Nicholas, 114
cystathione, 166
cysteine, 190
cytochrome P450 1A1, 178, 181
cytokines, 148, 149, 150, 155

dairy industry, 241–42
Denmark, 210
Dietary Supplement Health Education Act
    (1994), 98
diet books, 238–39
dill, 45, 116
DMBA, 176
DNA, xiv, xvi, xvii, 4–12, 40
    bases in, 4–5
    dietary protection of, 6–12, 18, 20, 43,
        79, 96, 97, 124, 142, 147
    double helix of, 5
    mitochondrial, 189, 190, 215–17
    mutations in, 141, 149, 166–67, 171–72,
        174, 177, 179, 189
    plant, mutations of, 221–22
    repair system of, 139, 140, 141, 143, 174,
        189
    telomeres, 188–89
    see also chromosomes; genes, genetic factors
DNA, damage to, 5–9, 87, 89, 92, 137–47,
        167, 175, 177, 184
    antioxidant defense system against, 138,
        139–41, 142–43
    in common diseases, 8–9, 138
    deadliness of, 141–42
    fats and, 144–46
    inflammation in, 143–47
    oxygen radicals in, 5–6, 8, 9, 16, 86, 96,
        137, 138–43, 150, 176–77, 189, 190,
        197, 209
    pollutants in, 140–41
    smoking in, 139–40, 143–44
dopamine, 206–7
Dorgan, Tad, 230
doughnuts, history of, 230
dressing, tofu, 65

eating behaviors, 201–12
    addictions and, 206–7
    binge eating, 208–9
    body fat set-point and, 210–11
    brain's pleasure center in, 206–7, 208
    carbohydrate cravings in, 207
    eating when not hungry, 203
    food choices in, 203, 204
    increased portion sizes, 206
    in infancy, 201–3
    monotonous diets and, 210, 212
    rushed eating, 203–4
    stress eating, 4, 124, 208
    sweeteners in, 204–5
    tastes in, 204–5, 209

    trigger foods in, 208
    see also overeating
echinacea, 98–99
egg white omelet with spinach, onion,
        mushrooms, tomatoes, and mixed
        herbs, 24, 30, 47, 64
Egyptians, ancient, 3, 102, 154, 222
eleutherosides, 101
ellagic acid, 180
endorphins, 120, 127
enzymes, 6–8, 18, 96, 111, 140–41, 161,
        166, 175, 178, 181, 188, 218
evolution, xvii, 3–4, 6, 9, 19, 95, 143, 172,
        208, 209, 213–14, 216, 218–20
    cholesterol in, 158–59, 161, 164
    inflammation in, 169
    malnutrition in, 153
    sex drive in, 195–96
    starvation adaptations in, 11, 153,
        154–55, 192
    see also hunter-gatherers; plant-based diet
evolution, cultural, 213–27, 228
    migrations in, 214–17
    see also agriculture; food industry
exercise, 12, 86–92, 151, 168
    eating before and after, 91–92
    fitness, 87–88
    as healthy addiction, 88
    muscle building, 86–87, 88–91
    stretching in, 88
    as sufficient for weight loss, 127–28
    target heart rate and, 88
    weight-bearing, 194
exercise equipment, 87–88
    calories burned by, 127–28
eye health, 15, 18, 187
    maintaining, 193–94

fat cells, 6, 148–56
    antioxidants stored in, 148, 150–51
    cytokines in, 148, 149, 150, 155
    distribution of, 151
    fertility related to, 154, 155
    functions of, 148, 151
    in immune system, 149, 150, 152
    inflammation and, 9, 149, 150
    leptin secreted by, 149, 150, 153, 154
    NPY levels and, 153
    number of, 151
    protective chemicals stored by, 148,
        150–51
    sex hormones related to, 148, 151,
        154–55

small babies and, 153
subcutaneous, 151–52
see also body fat
fats, xiv, xvi, 3, 10, 18, 20, 45, 79, 205, 231,
    242–43
    animal, 121, 145
    calories in, 121, 144
    cancer and, 182–83
    controlling intake of, 14–15
    desirable vs. undesirable, 18–19
    in DNA damage, 144–46
    eliminating, for weight loss, 125
    monounsaturated, 15, 41, 46, 108, 121,
        129, 144, 146
    in nuts, 120–21
    polyunsaturated, 15, 40–41, 121, 130,
        144–46
    removal of products containing, 40–41
    restaurants and, 77–78
    saturated, 121, 144, 146
fatty acids, 15, 40–41, 121, 131, 143, 155,
    169, 179, 182–83
fertility, 154, 155
feverfew, 99–100
fiber, xvi, 20, 40, 128, 169, 205
fibrinogen, 167–68
figs, 108–9
Finland, 155–56
fish oils, 131, 146, 164
flavonoids, 11, 18, 97, 120, 143
folic acid, 93, 94, 166–67, 178, 181, 201
food choices, 203, 204, 218–20, 242, 244
food industry, 204–5, 228–45
    academic community and, 240, 242
    consumer preferences met by, 219, 242–44
    dietary guidelines and, 240–41, 244–45
    dietary variety and, 238, 239–40, 242
    fat-free foods produced by, 242–43
    fusion cuisine and, 237–38
    government and, 229, 240–43
    history of, 228–33
    "junk" foods and, xiv, 19, 238
    marketing by, 219, 220, 228, 234–36,
        241–42
    processed foods of, 4, 10, 145, 214, 219,
        220, 237–38, 244
    taste modification by, 205
    weight-loss industries and, 238–40
    see also agriculture
fortune cookies, 78
Framingham study, 167
French fries, production of, 242
fresh fruit and yogurt sundae, 25, 31

Friedman, Jeff, 149
frozen foods, 43, 108, 132
fruit bowl, 26
fruit juice industry, 242
fusion cuisine, 223–24, 237–38

garlic, 45, 117
    as herbal supplement, 102
garlic allyl sulfides, 181
genes, genetic factors, xiii, 5, 6, 11, 15, 20,
        132, 138, 142, 149, 151, 171–72, 189,
        214–20, 225, 234
    in aging, 188–89, 192–93, 198
    in body fat distribution, 152, 211
    in cancer, 171–72, 173, 174, 177, 178–79,
        218
    in cholesterol levels, 159, 161–64
    in dopamine receptors, 206–7
    in eating behavior, *see* eating behaviors
    flexibility in, 234
    in heart disease, 157, 158, 161–67, 169,
        218
    in prescription drug tolerance, 218
    in racial differences, 215, 217, 218
    in tastes, 204–5
    variations in, 172, 178–79, 206–7,
        215–18, 235–36
    see also chromosomes; DNA
genistein, 181
genome, human, xvii, 141, 215, 218, 234,
    245
German Commission Monograph E, The,
    105
ginger, 45
ginkgo biloba, 102–3
ginkgo flavonoid glycosides, 103
ginseng, 101
glucosinolates, 181
glutathione, 96, 108, 166, 182, 190
grains, 3, 128, 237
    hybrid corn, 224
    in livestock feed, 145
    mutations in, 221–22
    whole, 20, 32, 37, 40, 46, 71, 74, 180
grapefruit juice, 7–8
Greek restaurants, 81
Greeks, ancient, 104, 109, 114, 116, 222
green group, 6, 15, 18, 36, 44, 79, 80, 114,
    180
    in men's diet plan, 26–31
    in women's diet plan, 21–25
green salad 23, 28
green tea, 12, 79, 96, 97, 142, 180

green tea extract capsules, 96, 97
guavas, 109

halibut and vegetable kabobs, 23, 29, 47,
  59–60
hamburger, history of, 231
Hawaiian smoothie, 29
heart attacks, 140, 145, 158, 160–61, 166,
  168, 170, 192
heart disease, 5, 8, 9, 11, 12, 13, 17, 99,
  125, 148, 150, 156, 157–70, 188, 193,
  209, 212, 241
  death rate from, 161
  diet in, 157, 158–60, 165, 166, 169
  fibrinogen in, 167–68
  genetic factors in, 157, 158, 161–67, 169,
  218
  homocysteine levels in, 160, 165–67
  infections in, 142, 168–69
  inflammation in, 142, 144, 160, 168–69
  oxygen radicals in, 138, 139, 141–42
  prevention of, 169, 170
  risk factors for, 159, 160, 164–65, 167, 218
  see also cholesterol
Helicobacter pylori, 142, 168
herbal supplements, 97–105
  Chinese red yeast rice, 99, 160
  echinacea, 98–99
  feverfew, 99–100
  garlic, 102
  ginkgo biloba, 102–3
  ginseng, 101
  kava kava, 103
  St. John's wort, 104–5
  saw palmetto, 100–101
  valerian, 104
herbs, 115–18, 225, 237
  basil, 116
  chives, 116
  dill, 45, 116
  growing one's own, 115
  mint, 116–17
  oregano, 45, 117
  parsley, 117
  rosemary, 45, 117–18
  sage, 118
  tarragon, 118
  thyme, 45, 118
Herpesvirus hominus, 168–69
high-protein diets, 12, 14, 239
  ketosis produced by, 127
holidays, 83–84
homocysteine, 160, 165–67

Hong Qu (red yeast rice), 99, 160, 163
hot dogs, 84
  history of, 230–31
hunter-gatherers, 11, 106, 172, 196, 206,
  211, 218–21, 233–35
hypercholesterolemia, type IIA, 161
hypericin, 104

ice cream, history of, 232–33
immune system, 98, 141, 142, 143–44, 168,
  169, 174, 190, 202
  fat cells in, 149, 150, 152
  leptin in, 149, 150
  macrophages of, 160
  pro-biotic bacteria in, 183–84
impotence, 196
India, 79–80, 102, 111, 222, 232
indoles, 18
infections, 98, 148, 149, 150, 155, 192, 193,
  202, 241, 244
  in cancer, 142
  in heart disease, 142, 168–69
  obesity and, 152
inflammation, xiii, 89, 97, 119, 143–47, 160
  in cancer, 144, 168, 183
  diet and, 144–46
  fat cells and, 9, 149, 150
  in heart disease, 142, 144, 160, 168–69
ipriflavone, 195
isothiocyanates, 18, 114, 181
Italian restaurants, 81

Japanese restaurants, 79
Jefferson, Thomas, 229, 232–33
Jews, 216–17
  Ashkenazi, 217
  Cohanim of, 216
  Lemba tribe and, 217
Jungle, The (Sinclair), 231

kabobs, halibut and vegetable, 23, 29, 47,
  59–60
kaempferol, 18
kava kava, 103
ketchup, history of, 231–32
ketosis, 127
King, Mary Claire, 215
kiwi fruits, 109–10
kumquats, 110
kwashiorkor, 202

Lappé, Frances Moore, 238
lean body mass, xvi, 14, 247–49

Leibel, Rudy, 149
Lemba, 217
lens dislocation, 165
leptin, 149, 150, 153, 154
limonoids, 163, 180
linoleic acid, 145–46, 155
linolenic acid, 155
liposuction, 151–52
liver, 18, 99, 151, 158–59, 163, 174, 190
    detoxification system of, 141, 143,
        177–78
lovastatin (mevinolin), 99, 163
lutein, 15, 18, 108, 142, 193–94, 198
lychee fruit, 110–11
lycopene, 15, 16, 43, 52, 118, 142, 231,
    243

McCully, Kilmer, 165–66
macular degeneration, xv, 15, 18, 187,
    193–94
malnutrition, 150, 152, 190, 191, 239, 244
    in utero, 153, 201
    see also starvation
mangoes, 111
margarine, 130
marigold, 194
marinated cucumber salad, 24, 30, 47, 68
Masai, 162
meat industry, 239
meditation, 12
memory loss, 103, 197–98
men, 10, 79, 100, 167, 172–73, 175, 192,
    195, 209, 245
    ancient migrations of, 216
    body fat distribution of, 155, 211
    diet plans for, 20, 26–38
    fertility of, 154
    hormonal changes in, 211
    optimal body fat percentage of, 155
    prostate gland of, 15, 100, 144
    sex drive in, 196
metformin (Glucophage), 155
methionine, 166–67, 178
mevinolin (lovastatin), 99, 163
Mexican restaurants, 80–81
micronutrients, 179–82
Middle Eastern restaurants, 81–82
migraine headaches, 99–100
milk, 41, 225, 241–42
    baby formula, 202–3
    breast, 202, 211
    fermentation of, 184
    fortified, 212

Mindell, Earl, 239
mint, 116–17
monacolins, 99
muscles, 12, 14, 86–87, 88–91, 92, 97, 126,
    128, 151, 191, 195, 211
myths, nutritional, 123–33
    bananas and carrots as fattening in, 129
    basic four food groups in, 128–29
    cheese crackers as calcium source in, 19,
        132
    cholesterol levels in, 130–31
    eating less in, 124
    eliminating fats in, 125
    eliminating sugar in, 125–26
    exercise in, 127–28
    frozen vs. fresh vegetables in, 132
    high-protein diets and ketosis in, 127
    margarine and vegetable oils in, 130
    peanut butter as protein source in, 129
    pork as white meat in, 130
    salmon in, 131
    shrimp in, 131
    starvation mode in, 126–27
    vitamin and mineral supplements in, 128–29
    weight loss in, 124–28

N-acetylcarnitine, 190
Native Americans, 98, 100–101, 224, 237
    in California, 220–21
    domestication by, 223
New Guinea, 4, 165
NPY levels, 153
nuts, 45, 46, 106, 120–21, 129, 180

oatmeal and eggs, 22, 27
obesity, xv, 8, 9, 11, 12, 130, 147, 161, 162,
    167, 190, 192, 207, 208, 209–10, 225,
    233
    as cancer risk factor, 179
    infectious diseases and, 152
    leptin as cure for, 149, 150
    small babies and, 153, 202
office parties, holiday, 84
Olestra, 229, 242–43
olive oil, 15, 41, 45, 46, 76, 144, 146, 222
omega-3 fatty acids, 41, 121, 131, 145, 146,
    169, 183
omega-6 fatty acids, 40–41, 131, 145–46,
    169, 183
omelet, egg white, with spinach, onion,
    mushrooms, tomatoes, and mixed
    herbs, 24, 30, 47, 64
open-face turkey/avocado sandwich, 22

orange-banana-strawberry soy protein
shake, 21, 26, 47, 48
orange group, 6, 17, 35, 44, 79, 80, 111,
113, 181
in men's diet plan, 26–31
in women's diet plan, 21–25
orange/yellow group, 17, 35, 44, 79, 80–81,
109, 110, 112, 114, 180
in men's diet plan, 26–31
in women's diet plan, 21–25
oregano, 45, 117
osteoporosis, 93, 187, 193, 194–95
overeating, 9, 150
control of, 10
disease risk increased by, 209
by small babies, 153, 202
as stimulated by variety, 209–10
see also eating behaviors
Owens, Kelly, 215
oxalate, 95
oxygen, 5–6, 86, 137–39, 177
oxygen poisoning, 137
oxygen radicals, xiv, 5–6, 8, 9, 16, 86, 96,
137, 138–43, 150, 159, 176–77, 189,
190, 197, 209

papayas, 17, 111
paprika, 119
parsley, 117
parsley oil capsules, 117
parthenolide, 99–100
passion fruit, 112
peanut butter, 129
history of, 232
peanuts, 46, 120, 129
pedometers, 87–88, 128, 251
peppermint, 116
peppers, 119–20
pernicious anemia, 167
Persian cuisine, 82
persimmons, 106, 112–13
phyllo dough, 82
phytochemicals, phytonutrients, xiv, 6–8, 7,
10–11, 15, 16–18, 19–20, 92, 106, 118,
132, 172, 180–82, 225–27
phytoestrogens, 194–95
phytosterols, 108, 158, 163, 169
pita pocket tuna sandwich, 24, 30, 47, 65
Pitts, Gary, 236
pizza snack, quick, 26
plant-based diet, xvii, 3–4, 80, 95, 105, 141,
143, 144, 145, 165, 166, 169, 172,
177, 178, 198

biodiversity and, 215, 217, 220–21, 227,
235–36
cholesterol in, 158–59, 161, 162, 164
plant evolution influenced by, 218–20
wild plants in, 218–21, 234–35
plant domestication, 222–23
plaques, arterial, 160–61, 168, 169
Polo, Marco, 232, 237
polycystic ovarian syndrome (PCO), 154–55
polyphenols, 96, 97, 180
pomegranates, 113–14, 222
popcorn, air-popped, 46
pork, 130, 224
potato chip, history of, 229
PPAR-gamma protein, 145–46
prednisone, 183
prescription drugs, tolerance of, 218
Pritikin, Nathan, 239
progeria, 189
prostaglandins, 145–46
protein, dietary, xvi, 12, 18, 20, 41, 87, 92,
120, 129, 218, 220–21
calculating requirement for, 14, 247–49
desirable vs. undesirable, 18–19
low-fat, 10
peanut butter as source of, 129
sources of, 33–34
soy, see soy protein
protein bars, 83
muscle-recovery, 92
pudding, quick tofu fruit, 28
pycnogenol, 97

quercetin, 18
quick pizza snack, 26
quick tofu fruit pudding, 28

recipes, 47–69
recommended dietary allowance (RDA),
94–95, 240–41
inadequacy of, 244–45
red group, 6, 16, 34, 44, 79, 80, 181
in men's diet plan, 26–31
in women's diet plan, 21–25
red/purple group, 16–17, 34–35, 44, 79, 80,
109, 111, 112, 114, 180
in men's diet plan, 26–31
in women's diet plan, 21–25
red yeast rice (Hong Qu), 99, 160, 163
restaurants, 39, 41, 45, 74, 75–83, 239
fats and, 77–78
guidelines for, 76
ordering in, 82

portion size in, 77, 206
see also specific ethnic restaurants
retrolental fibroplasia, 137
rice bran oil, 163
Roberts, Susan, 210
Romans, ancient, 3, 104, 116, 187, 222
rosemary, 45, 117–18
Rubin, David, 238–39

sage, 118
St. John's wort, 104–5
salad:
    chef's, with balsamic vinaigrette, 25, 31,
        47, 69
    chicken breast seven color, 21, 26, 47, 48–49
    chopped vegetable, 22, 28, 47, 54–55
    dressings, 14–15, 69, 76, 80, 82, 108
    green, 23, 28
    marinated cucumber, 24, 30, 47, 68
    tuna niçoise, 21, 27, 47, 51
salmon, 131
sandwich:
    turkey/avocado, 28
    turkey/avocado, open-face, 22
sautéed Swiss chard, 22, 27, 47, 54
saw palmetto, 100–101
seasonal affective disorder (SAD), 207
selenium, 96, 120
serotonin, 207
sex drive, 195–97
sex hormones, 148, 151, 154–55, 158,
    194–95, 196, 211
shakes, soy protein, 10, 25, 31
    orange-banana-strawberry, 21, 26, 47, 48
Shaw, George Bernard, 198
Shen Nung's Materia Medica, 101
shrimp, 10, 131
shrimp, tofu, and broccoli stir-fry, 21, 26,
    47, 49–50
slaw, cabbage and bell pepper, 23, 29, 47,
    57–58
smell, sense of, 219
smoking, 139–40, 143–44, 167, 168, 172,
    177–78, 206–7
smoothie:
    Hawaiian, 29
    soy, 27
snack foods, xiv–xv, 10, 15, 43–44, 125,
    132, 204, 205, 210, 243
    removal of, 39–40
soy:
    meat sauce, whole-wheat pasta with, 22,
        47, 56–57

nugget cereal with fruit, 21, 26
    smoothie, 27
soy isoflavones, 194–95
soy milk, 41, 52
soy protein, 10, 12, 14, 20, 45–46, 70, 73,
    79, 84, 142, 194–95, 231
soy protein shakes, 10, 25, 31
    orange-banana-strawberry, 21, 26, 47, 48
Spanish cuisine, 82
spices, 45, 99, 106, 119–20, 225
spicy fish stew, 24, 30, 47, 63
starfruit, 106, 114
starvation, 149, 201, 237
    adaptations to, 11, 153, 154–55, 192
starvation mode, 126–27
statin drugs, 163, 164
stew, spicy fish, 24, 30, 47, 63
stir-fry, shrimp, tofu, and broccoli, 21, 26,
    47, 49–50
stress eating, 4, 124, 208
sugar, xiv, 10, 12, 125–26, 147, 204–5, 212,
    243
sulforaphane, 18, 180, 182
sundae(s)
    fresh fruit and yogurt, 25, 31
    history of, 232–33
supplements, 11, 12, 19, 92, 93–105, 142,
    146, 177, 180, 239
    for aging, 190–91, 192, 193–94, 198
    basic four food groups and, 93, 95,
        128–29
    core group of, 94–98
    deficiencies and, 93
    legal right to, 98
    see also herbal supplements; vitamins and
        minerals
sweet-and-sour stuffed cabbage, 24, 30, 47,
    66–67
Swiss chard, sautéed, 22, 27, 47, 54
Szechuan cuisine, 78, 223

Tarahumara Indians, 162
target heart rate, 88, 127
tarragon, 118
taste enhancers, 20, 32, 38, 45, 46, 72, 74,
    109, 119–20, 121–22, 129, 146, 225,
    227
taste modification, 205
tastes, 204–5, 209, 218–19, 225, 228, 231,
    232, 233, 237–38, 243, 244
telomeres, 188–89
thyme, 45, 118
tocotrienols, 163

tofu, 45, 79, 84
  dressing, 65
  fruit pudding, quick, 28
tomatoes, tomato products, 15, 16, 17, 43,
    83, 107, 132, 231–32, 237, 243
tomato-soy bisque, 22, 27, 47, 52
traveling, 39, 75–85, 94
  guidelines for, 83
  see also restaurants
trigger foods, 208
triglycerides, 159, 160, 164–65
tuna:
  niçoise salad, 21, 27, 47, 51
  sandwich, pita pocket, 24, 30, 47, 65
turkey/avocado sandwich, 28
  open-face, 22

ubiquinone (coenzyme Q10), 97
USDA food pyramid, 220, 225–27, *226*

valerian, 104
vegetable oils, 12, 15, 40–41, 183, 212, 230
  as cholesterol lowering, 130
  in DNA damage, 144–46
vegetable salad, chopped, 22, 28, 47, 54–55
Venus of Willendorf, 154
vitamins and minerals, xvi, 11, 12, 93–97,
    132, 180–82, 190, 239
  A, 94, 119, 212
  B, 94, 164, 166–67
  B$_6$, 166–67
  B$_{12}$, 166–67, 192
  C, 6, 20, 94, 95, 113, 117, 119, 128, 139,
    142–43, 177, 190, 241
  copper, 94, 120
  D, 128, 158, 192, 212
  deficiencies of, 93, 167, 192, 201, 212,
    233, 241
  E, 92, 94, 95, 120, 128–29, 137, 139,
    142, 148, 150, 163, 177, 180, 190, 198
  folic acid, 93, 94, 166–67, 178, 181, 201
  selenium, 96, 120

  side effects of, 94
  zinc, 94, 120
  see also calcium

Walford, Roy, 190
watercress, 114
weightlifting, 86–87, 92
  circuit training in, 88–91
weight loss, 13–14, 120, 151–52, 155–56,
    168, 209, 210
  industries for, 238–40
  myths about, 124–28
white/green group, 18, 36–37, 44, 79, 80,
    81, 116, 181
  in men's diet plan, 26–31
  in women's diet plan, 21–25
whole-wheat:
  couscous, 22, 46
  pasta with soy meat sauce, 22, 28, 47,
    56
women, 10, 14, 79, 167, 172–73, 175, 192,
    209, 245
  ancient migrations of, 216
  body fat distribution in, 152, 211
  diet plans for, 20, 21–25, 32–38
  fertility of, 154, 155
  menopause of, 167, 196, 211
  optimal body fat percentage of, 155
  polycystic ovarian syndrome in, 154–55
  Scandinavian, 167
  sex drive in, 196

Y chromosome, 215–17
yellow/green group, 15, 18, 36, 44, 79, 80,
    81, 108, 110, 181, 193
  in men's diet plan, 26–31
  in women's diet plan, 21–25
yogurt, live-culture, 184

zeaxanthin, 15, 18, 193–94
zinc, 94, 120
Zone Diet, 129